T0200034

CASES IN
HOSPITAL
MEDICINE

An Evidence-Based Approach

CASES IN
HOSPITAL
MEDICINE

An Evidence-Based Approach

Zahir Kanjee, MD, MPH, FACP
Hospitalist and Clinician-Educator
Beth Israel Deaconess Medical Center
Instructor in Medicine
Harvard Medical School
Boston, Massachusetts

Joshua M. Liao, MD, MSc, FACP
Hospitalist and Clinician Scholar
Director, Value & Systems Science Lab
Assistant Professor
Department of Medicine
University of Washington School of Medicine
Seattle, Washington

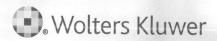. Wolters Kluwer

Philadelphia • Baltimore • New York • London
Buenos Aires • Hong Kong • Sydney • Tokyo

Acquisitions Editor: Sharon Zinner
Development Editor: Elizabeth Schaffer
Editorial Coordinator: Dave Murphy
Production Project Manager: Jaon Sinclair
Design Coordinator: Joseph Clark
Manufacturing Coordinator: Beth Welsh
Prepress Vendor: TNQ Technologies

Copyright © 2020Wolters Kluwer.

All rights reserved. This book is protected by copyright. No part of this book may be reproduced or transmitted in any form or by any means, including as photocopies or scanned-in or other electronic copies, or utilized by any information storage and retrieval system without written permission from the copyright owner, except for brief quotations embodied in critical articles and reviews. Materials appearing in this book prepared by individuals as part of their official duties as U.S. government employees are not covered by the above-mentioned copyright. To request permission, please contact Wolters Kluwer at Two Commerce Square, 2001 Market Street, Philadelphia, PA 19103, via email at permissions@lww.com, or via our website at shop.lww.com (products and services).

9 8 7 6 5 4 3 2 1

Printed in China

Library of Congress Cataloging-in-Publication Data

ISBN-13: 978-1-975111-57-1

Cataloging in Publication data available on request from publisher.

This work is provided "as is," and the publisher disclaims any and all warranties, express or implied, including any warranties as to accuracy, comprehensiveness, or currency of the content of this work.

This work is no substitute for individual patient assessment based upon healthcare professionals' examination of each patient and consideration of, among other things, age, weight, gender, current or prior medical conditions, medication history, laboratory data and other factors unique to the patient. The publisher does not provide medical advice or guidance and this work is merely a reference tool. Healthcare professionals, and not the publisher, are solely responsible for the use of this work including all medical judgments and for any resulting diagnosis and treatments.

Given continuous, rapid advances in medical science and health information, independent professional verification of medical diagnoses, indications, appropriate pharmaceutical selections and dosages, and treatment options should be made and healthcare professionals should consult a variety of sources. When prescribing medication, healthcare professionals are advised to consult the product information sheet (the manufacturer's package insert) accompanying each drug to verify, among other things, conditions of use, warnings and side effects and identify any changes in dosage schedule or contraindications, particularly if the medication to be administered is new, infrequently used or has a narrow therapeutic range. To the maximum extent permitted under applicable law, no responsibility is assumed by the publisher for any injury and/or damage to persons or property, as a matter of products liability, negligence law or otherwise, or from any reference to or use by any person of this work.

shop.lww.com

DEDICATION

To my colleagues, trainees, and patients for inspiring me to be a lifelong learner and teacher. To my family—especially my wife, children, siblings, and parents—for supporting me at every step.

Zahir Kanjee, MD, MPH

For Geraldine, Abigail, and Allison, who despite have little connection to evidence-based hospital medicine, are nonetheless my unwavering inspiration to continue learning, practicing, and teaching it.

Joshua M. Liao, MD, MSc

CONTRIBUTORS

Tyler J. Albert, MD
Hospital & Specialty Medicine
Puget Sound VA Health Care
  System
Seattle, Washington

David Arboleda, MD
Assistant Professor
Department of Medicine
University of California,
  San Francisco
San Francisco, California

Mara Bann, MD
Clinical Instructor
Department of Medicine
University of Washington School
  of Medicine
Seattle, Washington

Neal Biddick, MD
Hospitalist, Beth Israel Deaconess
  Medical Center
Instructor in Medicine, Harvard
  Medical School
Boston, Massachusetts

Jonathan Bortinger, MD
Hospitalist, Beth Israel Deaconess
  Medical Center
Instructor in Medicine, Harvard
  Medical School
Boston, Massachusetts

Katerina L. Byanova, MD, MS
Global Health Fellow, Beth Israel
  Deaconess Medical Center
Clinical Fellow in Medicine,
  Harvard Medical School
Boston, Massachusetts

Amanda Cooke, MD
Hospitalist, Beth Israel Deaconess
  Medical Center
Instructor in Medicine, Harvard
  Medical School
Boston, Massachusetts

Kirsten Courtade, MD
Hospitalist, Beth Israel Deaconess
  Medical Center
Instructor in Medicine, Harvard
  Medical School
Boston, Massachusetts

Neha Deshpande, MD
Clinical Instructor
Department of Medicine
University of Washington School
  of Medicine
Seattle, Washington

Rahul Ganatra, MD, MPH
Hospitalist, Beth Israel Deaconess
  Medical Center
Instructor in Medicine, Harvard
  Medical School
Boston, Massachusetts

Divya Gollapudi, MD
Clinical Assistant Professor
Department of Medicine
University of Washington School
  of Medicine
Seattle, Washington

Rachel Hensel, MD
Hospitalist, Beth Israel Deaconess
  Medical Center
Instructor in Medicine, Harvard
  Medical School
Boston, Massachusetts

Jonathan Hourmozdi, MD
Resident Physician
Department of Medicine
University of Washington School
  of Medicine
Seattle, Washington

Jennifer Hu, MD
Hospitalist, Beth Israel Deaconess
  Medical Center
Instructor in Medicine, Harvard
  Medical School
Boston, Massachusetts

Andrew Junkin, MD
Hospitalist, Beth Israel Deaconess
  Medical Center
Instructor in Medicine, Harvard
  Medical School
Boston, Massachusetts

Nicholas Kiefer, MD
Resident Physician, Beth Israel
  Deaconess Medical Center
Clinical Fellow in Medicine,
  Harvard Medical School
Boston, Massachusetts

Mehraneh Khalighi, MD
Clinical Assistant Professor
Department of Medicine
University of Washington School
  of Medicine
Seattle, Washington

Christopher Kim, MD, MBA
Associate Professor
Department of Medicine
University of Washington School
  of Medicine
Seattle, Washington

**Christopher P. Kovach, MD,
MSc**
Resident Physician
Department of Medicine
University of Washington School
  of Medicine
Seattle, Washington

Henry R. Kramer, MD
Hospitalist, University of Colorado
  Hospital
Assistant Professor of Medicine -
  Hospital Medicine, University
  of Colorado
Aurora, Colorado

Eric M. LaMotte, MD
Clinical Instructor
Department of Medicine
University of Washington School
  of Medicine
Seattle, Washington

Dawn Lei, MD
Resident Physician, Beth Israel
  Deaconess Medical Center
Clinical Fellow in Medicine,
  Harvard Medical School
Boston, Massachusetts

Cindy Lien, MD
Palliative Care Physician and
  Hospitalist, Beth Israel
  Deaconess Medical Center
Assistant Professor of Medicine,
  Harvard Medical School
Boston, Massachusetts

Joy J. Liu, MD
Resident Physician, Beth Israel
  Deaconess Medical Center
Clinical Fellow in Medicine,
  Harvard Medical School
Boston, Massachusetts

Leah Marcotte, MD
Clinical Assistant Professor
Department of Medicine
University of Washington School
  of Medicine
Seattle, Washington

Patrick Marcus, MD
Resident Physician
Department of Medicine
University of Washington School
  of Medicine
Seattle, Washington

Amrita Mukhopadhyay, MD
Resident Physician, Beth Israel
  Deaconess Medical Center
Clinical Fellow in Medicine,
  Harvard Medical School
Boston, Massachusetts

Elijah J. Mun, MD
Resident Physician
Department of Medicine
University of Washington School
  of Medicine
Seattle, Washington

Maya Narayanan, MD, MPH
Clinical Assistant Professor
Department of Medicine
University of Washington School
  of Medicine
Seattle, Washington

Maria Nardell, MD
Hospitalist, Beth Israel Deaconess
  Medical Center
Instructor in Medicine, Harvard
  Medical School
Boston, Massachusetts

Scott Navarett, MD
Hospitalist, Beth Israel Deaconess
  Medical Center
Instructor in Medicine, Harvard
  Medical School
Boston, Massachusetts

Lauren Noll, MD
Resident Physician
Department of Medicine
University of Washington School
  of Medicine
Seattle, Washington

Nicholas D. Patchett, MD
Hospitalist, Beth Israel Deaconess
  Medical Center
Instructor in Medicine, Harvard
  Medical School
Boston, Massachusetts

William Rusty Phillips, MD
Hospitalist, Beth Israel Deaconess
  Medical Center
Instructor in Medicine, Harvard
  Medical School
Boston, Massachusetts

Celeste Pizza, MD
Internal Medicine Physician U.S.
    Embassy Health Clinic New Delhi,
    India

Kristen M. Rogers, MD, MPH
Resident Physician
Department of Medicine
University of Washington School
    of Medicine
Seattle, Washington

Megan U. Roosen-Runge, MD, MPH
Acting Instructor
Department of Medicine
University of Washington School
    of Medicine
Seattle, Washington

Mala M. Sanchez, MD
Clinical Instructor
Department of Medicine
VA Puget Sound Health Care
    System
University of Washington School
    of Medicine
Seattle, Washington

Staci Saunders, MD
Resident Physician, Beth Israel
    Deaconess Medical Center
Clinical Fellow in Medicine,
    Harvard Medical School
Boston, Massachusetts

Shobha W. Stack, MD, PhD
Acting Instructor
Department of Medicine
University of Washington School
    of Medicine
Seattle, Washington

Michael Charles C. Tan, MD
Resident Physician
Department of Medicine
University of Washington School
    of Medicine
Seattle, Washington

Courtney Tuegel, MD
Resident Physician
Department of Medicine
University of Washington School
    of Medicine
Seattle, Washington

Anita Vanka, MD, FHM
Hospitalist, Beth Israel Deaconess
    Medical Center
Assistant Professor of Medicine,
    Harvard Medical School
Boston, Massachusetts

Joseph S. Wallins, MD, MPH
Department of Medicine
Massachusetts General Hospital
Boston, Massachusetts

Jonathan Wang, MD
Hospitalist, Beth Israel Deaconess
    Medical Center
Instructor in Medicine, Harvard
    Medical School
Boston, Massachusetts

Erin Wu, MD
Resident Physician
Department of Medicine
University of Washington School
    of Medicine
Seattle, Washington

Yilin Zhang, MD
Clinical Instructor
Department of Medicine
University of Washington School
    of Medicine
Seattle, Washington

PREFACE

The two of us—practicing hospitalists and educators with a deep passion for evidence-based medicine—designed this book for a broad range of readers and uses. It is applicable to clinicians at all levels, including student and resident trainees, advanced practice clinicians, and attending physicians. It is written for both clinicians and educators, for personal self-study, or for teaching. It can be read cover to cover, or as needed when topics come up in practice or educational settings.

The case method and topics were purposely selected. A case-based approach mirrors the way hospital-based clinicians think and work, increasing the book's clinical usefulness. Importantly, we also believe the case method is the most intuitive and enjoyable way to learn and teach to content.

We selected chapters and points of emphasis based on their frequency or salience to hospital medicine. Instead of spanning comprehensively from initial presentation through diagnosis and ultimate treatment in every case, we chose to feature common conditions and situations that our readers are likely to encounter in the practice of hospital medicine. For instance, chapters about chronic conditions emphasize acute exacerbations of disease—the most likely scenario in which hospital-based clinicians are likely to care for these patients.

Arriving at these scenarios and clinical decision points allowed us to move naturally to the evidence. We emphasize the use of evidence to guide practice because we know that this skill is fundamental to delivering excellent care. As such, the book attempts to feature key elements of existing literature, highlighting its strengths, weaknesses, caveats, interpretations, and applications.

In addition to clinical practice, our hope is that this volume will serve as a useful teaching aid for educators at all levels. By highlighting pertinent questions and succinctly describing key evidence to answer them, the case-based method can facilitate discussion between educators and trainees. As such, the book will be a useful resource on rounds or at the white board. Moreover, by familiarizing readers with some of the evidence that can help guide decisions, this volume will allow the clinical supervisor to model principles of evidence-based practice.

From the outset, we knew that our ability to achieve our goals in this volume would be predicated on the team we assembled to write it. We were very fortunate in that regard and able to engage individuals from Beth Israel Deaconess Medical Center/Harvard Medical School and the University of Washington School of Medicine—world-class institutions with a pool of exceptionally talented colleagues. The scope, framing, and detail of our content were further strengthened by review from experts at these outstanding clinical and educational centers.

This is why and how we created this book. We are proud of the hard work from so many that it represents. We are also proud because we believe it has the potential to be of great use to hospital-based clinicians and, ultimately, their patients.

Zahir Kanjee, MD, MPH

Joshua M. Liao, MD, MSc

ACKNOWLEDGMENTS

We are grateful for the thoughtful review and input from physician experts at Beth Israel Deaconess Medical Center/Harvard Medical School and the University of Washington School of Medicine.

At Beth Israel Deaconess Medical Center/Harvard Medical School: Sarah Berry, Tyler Berzin, Jonah Cohen, Joseph Feuerstein, Shoshana Herzig, Sandeep Kumar, Mary LaSalvia, Amber Moore, Simi Padival, Vilas Patwardhan, Matthew Ronan, Mandeep Sawhney, Partha Sinha, Conor Stack, Jennifer Stevens, Jordan Strom, Jonathan Waks, and John Wixted.

At the University of Washington School of Medicine: Rosemary Adamson, Chloe Bryson-Cahn, Başak Çoruh, Richard K. Cheng, Paul Cornia, Ted Gibbons, Zachary Goldberger, Joe C. Huang, George Ioannou, Ryan J. Kimmel, Carey H. Paine, and Kristen Patton.

TABLE OF CONTENTS

Figure Credits

Chapter 1

Unnumbered figure 1: Reprinted from Webb WR, Higgins CB. *Thoracic Imaging*. Philadelphia: Wolters Kluwer; 2014 with permission.

Chapter 6

Unnumbered figure 1: LifeART image copyright (c) 2020 Lippincott Williams & Wilkins. All rights reserved.

Chapter 14

Unnumbered figure 1: Reprinted from Müller NL, Franquet T, Lee KS, et al. *Imaging of Pulmonary Infections*. Philadelphia: Lippincott Williams & Wilkins; 2007 with permission.

Chapter 15

Unnumbered figure 1: Reprinted from Lily LS. *Pathophysiology of Heart Disease*. Philadelphia: Wolters Kluwer; 2015 with permission.

Chapter 17

Unnumbered figure 1: Reprinted from Caughey AB. *Cases & Concepts Step 1: Pathophysiology Review*. Philadelphia: Wolters Kluwer; 2009 with permission.

Chapter 18

Unnumbered figure 1: Reprinted from Webb WR, Higgins CB. *Thoracic Imaging*. Philadelphia: Wolters Kluwer; 2010 with permission.

Chapter 23

Unnumbered figure 1: Reprinted from Woods SL, et al. *Cardiac nursing*. Philadelphia: Wolters Kluwer, 2019 with permission.

Unnumbered figure 2: Reprinted from Zimetbaum PJ, Josephson ME. *Practical Clinical Electrophysiology*. Philadelphia: Wolters Kluwer; 2017 with permission.

Chapter 28

Unnumbered figure 1: Reprinted from Hartley P, Adamson J, Cunningham C, Embleton G, Romero-Ortuno R. Clinical frailty and functional trajectories in hospitalized older adults: a retrospective observational study. *Geriatr Gerontol Int*. 2017;17(7):1063-1068. Epub 2016 July 18 with permission from Wiley.

CHAPTER 1

SEPSIS

Nicholas Kiefer, MD,
William Rusty Phillips, MD

A 77-year-old woman is admitted from the ED with worsening productive cough for a few days. Her vitals are notable for T 101°F, HR 110 bpm, BP 88/56 mm Hg, and RR 24, and her pulse oximeter reads 89% on room air. Her labs and imaging are notable for WBC 15 K/μL, Cr 1.5 mg/dL, and CXR with a left lower lobe consolidation. You are concerned about sepsis and order intravenous fluid (IVF), blood cultures, and antibiotics. The nurse places a peripheral intravenous catheter (PIV) and asks if she can administer the antibiotics after the IVF completes in an hour.

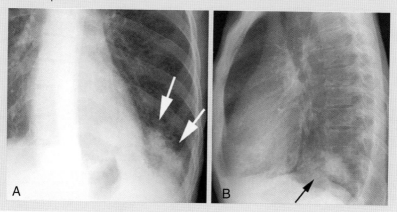

A   B

How soon should antibiotics be administered in the setting of possible sepsis?

Antibiotics should be administered as soon as there is a concern for sepsis.

A large retrospective analysis using the Surviving Sepsis Campaign (SSC) database was conducted in 2014 to determine the risk of mortality for delay in antibiotics in patients with severe sepsis and septic shock.[1] Authors reviewed charts of all patients from January 2005 to February 2010 at 165 ICUs in Europe, the United States, and South America. After excluding those without documented antibiotics or antibiotic timing as well as those already receiving antibiotics prior to presentation, the authors included 17,990 patients. A regression model was used to analyze the relationship between time to antibiotic administration and in-hospital mortality. The model controlled for ICU admission source, geographic location, and sepsis severity score.

The authors found that the adjusted mortality OR linearly increased each hour from 0 to 6 hours for time to antibiotic administration (using 0-1 hour as the referent group, $P < .05$ from 2 hours onward). A sample computation that used the ED as the admission source, the United States as the geographic location, and a sepsis severity score of 52 (median score for all observations) showed that the probability of mortality increased from 24.6% to 33.1% from a time of 0 hours to >6 hours. Caveats of this study include its retrospective nature as well as the lack of information about appropriateness of initial antibiotics.

> You ask the nurse to place another PIV and start antibiotics as soon as possible. As the fluids are infusing, you contemplate your resuscitation strategy.

Should patients with suspected septic shock receive resuscitation with early goal-directed therapy (EGDT)?

As a protocolized approach to sepsis management, EGDT does not reduce mortality compared to usual resuscitation.

EGDT is a protocolized approach for sepsis management utilizing arterial pressures, venous pressures, and $ScvO_2$ to guide administration

---

[1]Ferrer R, et al. Empiric antibiotic treatment reduces mortality in severe sepsis and septic shock from the first hour: results from a guideline-based performance improvement program. *Crit Care Med.* 2014;42(8):1749-1755.

of IVF, vasoactive agents, and blood transfusions.[2] In the original single-center randomized controlled trial, EGDT decreased short-term mortality compared to nonprotocolized management. This trial led to a major shift in practice whereby early and aggressive fluid resuscitation became the standard of care for sepsis. However, several subsequent large, high-quality trials comparing EGDT protocols to this new aggressive "usual care" have not shown the same benefit, bringing the utility of EGDT into question.

A 2015 systematic review and meta-analysis sought to more formally answer this question and compared EGDT to usual care in patients with septic shock who presented to the ED.[3] The authors performed a comprehensive literature review without language restrictions from 2000 to 2015 identifying randomized controlled trials of EGDT in septic shock. The primary outcome of interest was mortality; secondary outcomes were ICU admission rate, length of stay, and use of organ-supporting devices and medications. Eleven trials comprising 5407 patients were eventually included in the study.

EGDT did not decrease mortality in comparison to usual care (23.2% vs. 22.4%, pooled OR 1.01, 95% CI 0.88-1.16; $P = .90$). Patients receiving EGDT were more likely to receive vasopressors (pooled OR 1.25, 95% CI 1.10-1.41; $P < .001$) and be admitted to the ICU (pooled OR 2.19, 95% CI 1.82-2.65; $P < .001$). There was no difference in ICU length of stay (weighted mean difference −0.02 days, 95% CI −0.47 to 0.43; $P = .93$) or hospital length of stay (weighted mean difference −0.28 days, 95% CI −1.18 to 0.62; $P = .55$).

Overall, this meta-analysis concluded there was no evidence that EGDT improved outcomes. As a result, the 2016 SSC guidelines no longer recommend EGDT for resuscitation in sepsis.[4] Instead, the SSC recommends aggressive initial resuscitation with 30 mL/kg of IVF for the average patient with septic shock (based on the mean volume of IVF given pre-randomization in EGDT trials; strong recommendation, low quality of evidence).

> You administer 2 L of IVF but the patient's BP remains low at 84/58 mm Hg. You decide that she needs blood pressure support with vasoactive medications.

---

[2]Rivers E, et al. Early goal-directed therapy in the treatment of severe sepsis and septic shock. *N Engl J Med.* 2001;345(19):1368-1377.

[3]Angus DC, et al. A systematic review and meta-analysis of early goal-directed therapy for septic shock: the ARISE, ProCESS, and ProMISe investigators. *Intensive Care Med.* 2015;41(9):1549-1560.

[4]Rhodes A, et al. Surviving sepsis campaign: International guidelines for management of sepsis and septic shock: 2016. *Crit Care Med.* 2017;43(3):486-552.

Which vasoactive medication should be used first for a hypotensive patient with septic shock refractory to IVF?

Norepinephrine is the initial vasoactive medication of choice for septic shock.

A systematic review and meta-analysis examined 32 randomized controlled trials that compared norepinephrine with either dopamine, epinephrine, vasopressin/terlipressin, or phenylephrine in adults with septic shock.[5] The primary outcome was 28-day mortality, and secondary outcomes included ICU length of stay and adverse events (myocardial infarction, arrhythmias, cerebrovascular accident, skin necrosis, and internal organ ischemic damage).

Norepinephrine was associated with lower all-cause mortality compared to dopamine (RR 0.89, 95% CI 0.81-0.98; P = .02) but not compared to epinephrine (RR 0.96, 95% CI 0.77-1.21; P-value not reported), vasopressin/terlipressin (RR 1.07, 95% CI 0.91-1.26; P-value not reported), or phenylephrine (RR 0.92, 95% CI 0.64-1.32; P-value not reported). There were no differences between norepinephrine and other vasopressors in terms of length of stay in the ICU (mean difference 1.01 days, 95% CI −0.65 to 2.66; P-value not reported). Major adverse events were lower with norepinephrine in comparison to dopamine (RR 0.34, 95% CI 0.14-0.84; P-value not reported), especially for arrhythmias (RR 0.48, 95% CI 0.40-0.58; P-value not reported).

Study limitations include analysis of trials conducted from 1989 to 2012, during which great advances in sepsis management have occurred, as well as significant heterogeneity across included studies in regard to dosing, time to events, and monitoring.

The SSC recommends that norepinephrine should be the first-choice vasopressor in septic shock (strong recommendation, moderate quality of evidence), although acknowledges that most evidence supports norepinephrine over dopamine and that more studies need to be conducted on other vasopressors.[6]

---

[5]Avni T, et al. Vasopressors for the treatment of septic shock: Systematic review and meta-analysis. *PLoS One*. 2015;10:e01293505.
[6]See footnote 4.

The patient is started on norepinephrine and attains an adequate blood pressure. She is still tachypneic and becomes less responsive. She is admitted to the ICU for septic shock. As you are transferring the patient, the family asks if their loved one has "sepsis" and if she will recover.

What is the role of the systemic inflammatory response syndrome (SIRS) criteria, sequential organ failure assessment (SOFA), and the newer quick SOFA (qSOFA) in the diagnosis and prognosis of sepsis?

An infection-related increase in SOFA score ≥2 has replaced the previously used combination of SIRS criteria and suspected infection in the clinical definition of sepsis. Outside of the ICU, qSOFA criteria are emphasized as a key early predictor of sepsis-related mortality. While qSOFA criteria appear slightly better than SIRS for predicting in-hospital mortality, they are not clearly superior to SIRS for sepsis diagnosis.

SIRS criteria have traditionally been used in the diagnosis and prognostication of sepsis. Many authors have criticized SIRS for lacking both sensitivity (because of a focus on inflammation to the exclusion of other severe responses to infection) and specificity (because the criteria may be present in those without life-threatening infection) for sepsis diagnosis. Describing sepsis as "life-threatening organ dysfunction caused by a dysregulated host response to infection," the SSC recently replaced SIRS with SOFA—an organ dysfunction scoring system commonly used in ICUs, see Table 1.1—in the clinical definition of sepsis.[7]

Recognizing that SOFA was not well-known or used outside of the ICU and that its computation is complex and requires laboratory and physiologic values that may not be immediately available to providers, authors attempted to develop a simpler and more readily available scoring system to identify those at high risk for sepsis-related mortality. The qSOFA score was developed, and its ability to accurately predict

[7]Singer M, et al. The Third International Consensus Definitions for Sepsis and Septic Shock (Sepsis-3). *J Am Med Assoc.* 2016;315(8):801-810.

TABLE 1.1

Scoring Systems

Scoring System	Criteria
Systemic inflammatory response syndrome (SIRS)	≥2 of the following: 1. T >38 or <36°C 2. HR >90/min 3. RR >20/min or $PaCO_2$ <32 mm Hg 4. WBC >12000/mm³ or <4000/mm³ or >10% immature bands
Sequential organ dysfunction assessment (SOFA)	Acute increase in score ≥2 points due to infection: 1. Lung (0-4 points) 2. Coagulation (0-4 points) 3. Liver (0-4 points) 4. Cardiovascular (0-4 points) 5. Brain (0-4 points) 6. Kidney (0-4 points)
Quick sequential organ dysfunction assessment (qSOFA)	≥2 of the following: 1. Altered mental status 2. Systolic BP (SBP) ≤100 mm Hg 3. RR ≥22/min

SIRS data from Bone RC, et al. Definitions for sepsis and organ failure guidelines for the use of innovative therapies in sepsis. *Chest.* 1992;101(6):144-1655; qSOFA reprinted from Singer M, et al. The Third International Consensus Definitions for Sepsis and Septic Shock (Sepsis-3). *J Am Med Assoc.* 2016;315(8):801-810 with permission. Additional data from Rhodes A, et al. Surviving Sepsis Campaign: International Guidelines for Management of Sepsis and Septic Shock 2016. *Crit Care Med.* 45(3):486-552.

Note that qSOFA score selected by SSC guidelines is simplified, with "altered mental status" replacing Glasgow Coma Scale (GCS) ≤13.

mortality tested against that of SIRS and several existing organ dysfunction scoring systems (SOFA, logistic organ dysfunction system [LODS]), in a 2016 retrospective cohort study.[8]

The analysis utilized a primary cohort of 148,907 patients from 12 community and academic hospitals in Pennsylvania from 2010 to 2012. This population was divided into approximately equally sized derivation and validation cohorts. Four additional, external cohorts totaling 706,399 patients included all patients from 20 Northern California hospitals from 2009 to 2013, all patients from 130 Veterans Affairs

---

[8]Seymour CW, et al. Assessment of clinical criteria for sepsis. *J Am Med Assoc.* 2016;315(8): 762-774.

hospitals from 2008 to 2010, all patients from a German hospital with hospital-acquired infections who were enrolled in a prior cohort study from 2011 to 2012, and all nontrauma and nonarrest patients from five advanced life support agencies in Washington from 2009 to 2010. Patients were deemed to have infection based on medical records showing orders for both antibiotics and cultures. The authors derived the qSOFA (two out of three of GCS ≤13, SBP ≤100 mm Hg, and RR ≥22/min) using univariate logistic regression on the derivation cohort. They then compared the discrimination of mortality (expressed as area under the receiver operating curve [AUROC]) between SOFA, qSOFA, SIRS, and LODS in the validation cohort. For patients in the ICU, SOFA (AUROC = 0.74) was superior at discriminating hospital mortality to qSOFA (AUROC = 0.66; $P < .001$), which in turn was superior to SIRS (AUROC = 0.64; $P = .01$). For patients outside the ICU, qSOFA outperformed both SIRS and SOFA at discriminating hospital mortality (AUROC = 0.81; $P < .001$ for both comparisons). Similar results were obtained in the external cohorts.

In light of these findings, in 2016, the SSC recommended qSOFA (substituting altered mental status for GCS ≤13 given a sensitivity analysis that showed this simplification did not have any meaningful effect on performance) be used "to identify adult patients with suspected infection who are likely to have poor outcomes" and "prompt clinicians to further investigate for organ dysfunction (such as the full SOFA criteria), to initiate or escalate therapy as appropriate, and to consider referral to critical care."[9]

Others have subsequently sought to study and compare qSOFA and SIRS in other populations, both for mortality discrimination as well as predicting sepsis. A 2018 systematic review and meta-analysis[10] included 10 observational studies accounting for 229,480 prehospital, ED, ward, and ICU patients. The AUROC for hospital mortality of qSOFA was found to be slightly superior to that of SIRS (RR 0.03, 95% CI 0.01-0.05; $P = .002$). In terms of sepsis diagnosis, SIRS was found to be more sensitive (RR 1.32, 95% CI 0.40-2.24; $P < .0001$) but less specific (84.4%, 95% CI 76.2%-90.6% vs. 97.3%, 95% CI 92.1%-99.4%; P-value not reported) than qSOFA. Study limitations include variability in defining infection, high heterogeneity in several findings (I^2 ranging

---

[9]See footnote 7.

[10]Serafim R, et al. A comparison of the quick-SOFA and systemic inflammatory response criteria for the diagnosis of sepsis and the prediction of mortality: A systematic review and meta-analysis. *Chest*. 2018;153(3):646-655.

48%-100%), over 80% of the total patients in the meta-analysis being accounted for by one large cohort, and use of diagnostic specificity findings based on results from only one study.

In summary, the 2016 SSC guidelines[11] recommend qSOFA to identify those at risk of developing sepsis, a condition now diagnosed formally with an infection and elevated SOFA score. While qSOFA is slightly more discriminant than SIRS for predicting hospital mortality, it is also less sensitive than SIRS for the development of sepsis.

> Recognizing that she has infection-related organ dysfunction with an increase in her SOFA score, you confirm that the patient has sepsis. Noting the qSOFA score, you also state that her mortality risk is elevated.

KEY LEARNING POINTS

1. Antibiotics should be administered as soon as there is a concern for sepsis.
2. As a protocolized approach to sepsis management, EGDT does not reduce mortality compared to usual resuscitation.
3. Norepinephrine is superior to dopamine and is the initial vasoactive medication of choice for septic shock.
4. An infection-related increase in SOFA score ≥2 has replaced the previously used combination of SIRS criteria and suspected infection in the clinical definition of sepsis. Outside of the ICU, qSOFA criteria are emphasized as a key early predictor of sepsis-related mortality. While qSOFA criteria appear slightly better than SIRS for predicting in-hospital mortality, they are not clearly superior to SIRS for sepsis diagnosis.

---

[11]See footnote 7.

ACUTE PANCREATITIS

Katerina L. Byanova, MD, MS

A 60-year-old female patient presents to the ED with a 1-day history of nausea, vomiting, and sharp abdominal pain radiating to her back. On examination, she has epigastric tenderness and guarding. Workup reveals idiopathic acute pancreatitis, and you admit the patient to the medicine service. On arrival to the floor, her vitals are T 99.6°F, BP 110/60 mm Hg, HR 110 bpm, RR 20. You consider the best approach to crystalloid resuscitation.

What is the preferred strategy for intravenous fluid (IVF) administration in early acute pancreatitis?

Early fluid resuscitation improves outcomes in acute pancreatitis. Lactated Ringer's (LR) may be a better fluid choice than normal saline (NS).

A retrospective cohort study[1] of 434 patients presenting with acute pancreatitis to a single tertiary medical center over 24 years looked at the optimal timing of IVF administration. Included were patients who presented directly to the medical center and whose primary admission diagnosis was acute pancreatitis. Patients were excluded if the IVF they received was incompletely documented. Using nursing administration documentation, patients were divided into "early" (receiving >1/3 of the total 72-hour fluid volume within the first 24 hours, 340 patients) and "late" (receiving <1/3 of the total 72-hour fluid volume within the first 24 hours, 94 patients) resuscitation groups. Groups

---

[1]Warndorf MG, et al. Early fluid resuscitation reduces morbidity among patients with acute pancreatitis. *Clin Gastroenterol Hepatol.* 2011;9(8):705-709.

were well-balanced other than the early group having a lower proportion of patients who had post-ERCP (endoscopic retrograde cholangiopancreatography) acute pancreatitis (5% vs. 12%; $P = .03$) and were on TPN (26% vs. 46%; $P = .01$). Main outcomes included systemic inflammatory response syndrome (SIRS) or organ failure rates at 24, 48, and 72 hours, ICU transfers, duration of hospitalization, and mortality.

SIRS rates were comparable on admission but subsequently significantly lower in the early resuscitation group at all time points (24 hour: 15% vs. 32%, $P = .001$; 48 hour: 14% vs. 33%, $P = .001$; 72 hour: 10% vs. 23%, $P = .01$). Organ failure rates trended toward a difference only at 72 hours (5% vs. 10%; $P = .05$). Each of these differences persisted on multivariate adjustment. Length of stay (8 vs. 11 days; $P = .01$) and ICU transfer rates (6% vs. 17%; $P = .001$) were also lower in the early resuscitation group. Mortality rates did not differ (3% vs. 4%; $P = .70$). While the early resuscitation group received more IVF than the late group in the first 24 hours (mean 3.4 vs. 2.4 L; $P = .001$), they received less total fluid in the first 72 hours (mean 7.6 vs. 9.5 L; $P = .003$). Study caveats include confounding by indication, the lack of adjustment for secular trends, and the possibility of persistent unmeasured confounders.

A randomized controlled trial at three tertiary centers[2] compared goal-directed fluid resuscitation to standard therapy, in addition to use of LR versus NS, in 40 acute pancreatitis patients. Patients identified within 6 hours of initial presentation were included. Exclusion criteria were renal, cardiac, or liver disease, recent cardiovascular procedure or active chest pain, chronic obstructive pulmonary disease on home oxygen, active sepsis, electrolyte derangements, inflammatory diseases, cancer, or initial presentation to an outside hospital.

Patients were randomized to one of four treatment arms: goal-directed resuscitation with LR, goal-directed resuscitation with NS, standard resuscitation with LR, or standard resuscitation with NS. Goal-directed resuscitation consisted of following an algorithm of initial bolus and infusion with clinical reevaluation and blood urea nitrogen checks every 8 hours to assess fluid responsiveness, while standard resuscitation consisted of IVF given at the discretion of the treating physician. The primary outcome was presence of SIRS at 24 hours, while the secondary outcomes included serum CRP at 24 hours.

[2]Wu BU, et al. Lactated Ringer's solution reduces systemic inflammation compared with saline in patients with acute pancreatitis. *Clin Gastroenterol Hepatol.* 2011;9(8):710-717.

SIRS prevalence was lower than expected across all groups, leading to an underpowered primary outcome. Authors found that the goal-directed and standard resuscitation groups received similar amounts of fluid and that these strategies were not associated with any differences in SIRS or CRP at 24 hours. As compared to NS, use of LR led to lower rates of SIRS (84% vs. 0% relative reduction; P = .035) and CRP levels (51.5 vs. 104 mg/L; P = .02) at 24 hours.

A subsequent trial[3] showed improvement in various inflammatory markers with LR over NS without any notable side effects. Both of these studies are limited by stringent exclusion criteria, small sample sizes, and surrogate outcomes. The 2013 ACG guidelines[4] recommend early aggressive fluid resuscitation (strong recommendation, moderate quality of evidence), preferably with LR over NS (conditional recommendation, moderate quality of evidence), for patients without significant comorbidities such as renal or cardiac disease. The 2018 AGA guidelines[5] suggest goal-directed resuscitation (conditional recommendation, very low quality of evidence) and make no recommendation about choice of crystalloid.

> You initiate fluid resuscitation with LR. Evaluation for etiology is unrevealing, and over the next several days, the patient is not able to tolerate oral intake. You want to provide nutrition but are unsure which route is best.

What is the optimal route for providing nutrition in acute pancreatitis patients unable to tolerate oral intake?

Enteral nutrition (EN) improves morbidity and mortality compared to total parenteral nutrition (TPN).

This question was addressed by a 2010 systematic review[6] of eight randomized controlled trials representing a total of 348 adults with acute pancreatitis regardless of severity. Outcomes of interest included relative

---

[3]De-Madaria E, et al. Fluid resuscitation with lactated Ringer's solution vs normal saline in acute pancreatitis: a triple-blind, randomized, controlled trial. *United European Gastroenterol J.* 2017;6(1):63-72.

[4]Tenner S, et al. American College of Gastroenterology guideline management of acute pancreatitis. *Am J Gastroenterol.* 2013;108(9):1400-1415.

[5]Crockett SD, et al. American Gastroenterological Association Institute Guideline on initial management of acute pancreatitis. *Gastroenterology.* 2018;154(4):1096-1101.

[6]Al-Omran M, et al. Enteral versus parenteral nutrition for acute pancreatitis. *Cochrane Database Syst Rev.* 2010;(1):CD002837.

risk of death, multiple organ failure, systemic infections, need for surgery, local infections, and local noninfectious complications. Nonrandomized studies, trials that did not measure outcomes of interest, and trials in which patients were exposed to both TPN and EN were excluded.

EN was superior to TPN for risk of death (RR 0.50, 95% CI 0.28-0.91; P = .02), multiple organ failure (RR 0.55, 95% CI 0.37-0.81; P = .003), need for surgery (RR 0.44, 95% CI 0.29-0.67; P = .0001), and systemic infections (RR 0.39, 95% CI 0.23-0.65; P = .0003). Of note, findings were not statistically significant for rates of local infection (RR 0.74, 95% CI 0.40-1.35 P = .32), other local complications (RR 0.70, 95% CI 0.43-1.13; P = .15), length of hospital stay (−2.37 d, 95% CI −7.18 to −2.44; P = .33), and SIRS incidence (RR 1.00, 95% CI 0.17-5.89; P = 1.00). Caveats to this review include limited reporting of statistical data by some of the included trials, and small sample size.

These findings align with 2018 AGA guidelines,[7] which recommend EN over TPN for acute pancreatitis for those unable to tolerate oral intake (strong recommendation, moderate evidence).

> An enteral tube is placed and EN is initiated. Despite appropriate fluid resuscitation, the patient's abdominal pain and lab abnormalities persist and the disease progresses to severe acute pancreatitis. Knowing that infectious complications are a major cause of morbidity and mortality in severe acute pancreatitis patients, you consider starting prophylactic antibiotics.

Should patients with severe acute pancreatitis receive prophylactic antibiotics?

Severe acute pancreatitis patients should not receive prophylactic antibiotics.

A 2011 meta-analysis[8] assessed this question by evaluating a total of 841 patients from 14 randomized controlled trials that studied intravenous antibiotic prophylaxis versus placebo or supportive care in patients with severe (defined by several validated tools or CRP >120 mg/L) acute pancreatitis. The primary outcome was mortality, while secondary outcomes included incidence of infected necrosis, nonpancreatic infection, and need for surgery.

---

[7]See footnote 5.
[8]Wittau M, et al. Systematic review and meta-analysis of antibiotic prophylaxis in severe acute pancreatitis. *Scand J Gastroenterol.* 2011;46(3):261-270.

Antibiotic prophylaxis did not significantly reduce mortality (RR 0.74, 95% CI 0.50-1.07; $P = .11$), infected necrosis (RR 0.78, 95% CI 0.60-1.02; $P = .07$), nonpancreatic infection (RR 0.70, 95% CI 0.46-1.06; $P = .10$), or need for surgery (RR 0.93, 95% CI 0.72-1.20; $P = .58$). These results were confirmed in analysis including only the three double-blinded trials.

Study limitations include inclusion of patients with presumed pancreatic necrosis without contrast-enhanced CT confirmation, variation in timing of antibiotic prophylaxis (which ranged 1.5-5 days from presentation), and failure to stratify or control for size of pancreatic necrosis. Finally, many trials were not double-blinded and therefore at risk of bias.

These findings reflect 2018 AGA guidelines,[9] which advise against antibiotic prophylaxis for severe acute pancreatitis (conditional recommendation, low quality of evidence).

> You do not administer antibiotics. Over the next several days, the patient's pain and lab abnormalities begin to resolve and she is eventually able to tolerate adequate oral intake. She is discharged with primary care physician and gastroenterology follow-up.
>
> The next day, you admit another patient with acute pancreatitis. She is a 40-year-old overweight female with no medical history who presented to the ED with epigastric pain, vomiting, and elevated lipase. Right upper quadrant ultrasound shows cholelithiasis without choledocholithiasis, and the rest of the workup for causes of pancreatitis is unremarkable. You diagnose her with mild acute gallstone pancreatitis and start IVF. Her labs and clinical findings improve significantly over the next 36 hours. You consider whether to consult surgery for a cholecystectomy on this admission or to have her see a surgeon as an outpatient.

Is it preferable to perform cholecystectomy during the index admission for mild acute gallstone pancreatitis or to defer until outpatient follow-up?

For patients with mild acute gallstone pancreatitis, cholecystectomy during the index admission reduces complications without increasing surgical risk compared to a deferred procedure.

---

[9]See footnote 5.

PONCHO[10] was a randomized controlled trial comparing cholecystectomy timing in 266 adult patients with mild acute gallstone pancreatitis at 23 Dutch medical centers. Patients were included if they were thought to be approaching discharge (<48 hour), had CRP<100 mg/L, no longer required opioid medications, and were tolerating a regular oral diet. Those with advanced systemic disease (based on ASA class IV [severe systemic disease that is a constant threat to life] or, if >75 years old, ASA class III [severe systemic disease]), chronic pancreatitis, or ongoing alcohol abuse were excluded.

Patients in the index cholecystectomy group underwent the procedure ≤3 days from randomization, while those in the interval group were scheduled for cholecystectomy within 25 to 30 days. The primary outcome was a composite of readmission for biliary complications (pancreatitis, cholangitis, cholecystitis, choledocholithiasis requiring intervention, biliary colic) or death within 6 months. Secondary outcomes included individual components of the primary outcome, surgeon-rated difficulty of cholecystectomy on a 10-point scale, conversion to open procedure, and surgical complications.

The primary outcome occurred in fewer patients in the index group (5% vs. 17%, RR = 0.28, 95% CI 0.12-0.66; P = .002), a finding driven largely by lower rates of recurrent pancreatitis (2% vs. 9%, RR 0.27, 95% CI 0.08-0.92; P = .03). Neither difficulty of cholecystectomy (6/10 vs. 6/10; P = .70), conversion to open cholecystectomy (3% vs. 4%; P = .74), cystic duct leakage (1% vs. 1%; P = 1.00), nor bleeding requiring reoperation or transfusion (1% vs. 1%; P = 1.00) differed across groups.

Caveats are inclusion and exclusion criteria that may have selected for a particularly low-risk study population, and the low rate of surgical complications, which may limit ability to detect a meaningful difference in operative outcomes. Citing this trial, 2018 AGA guidelines[11] recommend cholecystectomy during index admission for patients with mild acute gallstone pancreatitis (strong recommendation, moderate quality of evidence).

> The patient undergoes uncomplicated laparoscopic cholecystectomy on hospital day 3 and is discharged 2 days later.

---

[10]Da Costa DW, et al. Same-admission versus interval cholecystectomy for mild gallstone pancreatitis (PONCHO): a multicentre randomised controlled trial. *Lancet.* 2015;386(1000):1261-1268.

[11]See footnote 5.

KEY LEARNING POINTS

1. Early fluid resuscitation improves outcomes in acute pancreatitis. LR may reduce inflammation more than NS and so may be a superior fluid choice.
2. EN improves morbidity and mortality compared to TPN in acute pancreatitis.
3. Severe acute pancreatitis patients should not receive prophylactic antibiotics as these medications do not reduce mortality or improve outcomes.
4. For patients with mild acute gallstone pancreatitis, cholecystectomy during the index admission reduces complications without increasing surgical risk compared to a deferred procedure.

SKIN AND SOFT TISSUE INFECTION

Neal Biddick, MD,
David Arboleda, MD

Overnight, you are called to assess a 63-year-old man admitted earlier in the day for a heart failure exacerbation who now complains of left forearm pain and redness. On physical examination, he is well-appearing and has an ill-defined area of erythema on his left forearm that is swollen and tender but without fluctuance or drainage. You diagnose the patient with cellulitis without abscess and decide to begin empiric antibiotics. You consider whether you should select antibiotics to cover him for methicillin-resistant *Staphylococcus aureus* (MRSA).

Do empiric antibiotics for cellulitis without abscess need to cover MRSA?

In patients with cellulitis without abscess, empiric MRSA coverage does not significantly increase clinical cure rates as compared with empiric *Streptococcus* coverage alone.

In a randomized double blinded trial conducted at three EDs in a MRSA-endemic area, 153 immunocompetent patients diagnosed in the outpatient setting with cellulitis without abscess and <1 week of symptoms were randomized to either cephalexin and trimethoprim-sulfamethoxazole (TMP-SMX) or cephalexin and placebo.[1] Exclusion criteria included current use of antibiotics, renal insufficiency, need for inpatient admission, immunocompromised state, indwelling catheter, peripheral vascular

---

[1]Pallin DJ, et al. Clinical trial: comparative effectiveness of cephalexin plus trimethoprim-sulfamethoxazole versus cephalexin alone for treatment of uncomplicated cellulitis: a randomized controlled trial. *Clin Infect Dis.* 2013;56(12):1754-1762.

disease complicating the cellulitis, bites, marine or freshwater injury, and diabetes. Patients were treated for a minimum of 7 days and told to continue antibiotics until 3 days after they felt "cured," to a maximum of 14 days. The primary outcome was clinical cure (defined as resolution of symptoms other than slight residual erythema or edema, and distinct from patient-assessed "cure" above) assessed at 12 and 30 days.

There was no difference in clinical cure across groups (85% in the cephalexin/TMP-SMX group vs. 82% in the cephalexin/placebo group, risk difference 2.7%, 95% CI, −9.3% to 15%; $P = .66$). There was no association between clinical cure and either nasal MRSA colonization status or purulence at enrollment (as defined by pustules <3 mm). Caveats include limited generalizability to the inpatient population and the exclusion of diabetics, who are at risk for polymicrobial infections.

These findings were supported by a subsequent double-blinded randomized trial of 496 patients at five US EDs that also compared cephalexin/TMP-SMX to cephalexin/placebo.[2] Inclusion and exclusion criteria were roughly similar to the study above, but this trial included diabetics (excluding diabetic foot infections). The primary outcome was clinical cure. The study used the absence of a series of failure criteria over 21 days including fever, erythema, swelling, and tenderness to define clinical cure.

Clinical cure occurred in a similar proportion of patients in each group (83.5% in the cephalexin/TMP-SMX group vs. 85.5% in the cephalexin/placebo group, risk difference −2.0%, 95% CI −9.7% to 5.7%; $P = .50$).

IDSA guidelines recommend against empiric antibiotics targeting MRSA for most cases of cellulitis in the absence of penetrating trauma, purulent drainage, active MRSA elsewhere on the body, known MRSA nasal colonization, injection drug use, or systemic inflammatory response syndrome (strong recommendation, moderate evidence).[3]

> Forgoing empiric MRSA coverage, you start the patient on cephalexin alone. He asks how long he needs to take this course of antibiotics.

[2]Moran GJ, et al. Effect of cephalexin plus trimethoprim-sulfamethoxazole vs cephalexin alone on clinical cure of uncomplicated cellulitis: a randomized clinical trial. *J Am Med Assoc.* 2017;317(20):2088-2096.

[3]Stevens DL, et al. Practice guidelines for the diagnosis and management of skin and soft tissue infections: 2014 update by the Infectious Disease Society of America. *Clin Infect Dis.* 2014;59(2):10-52.

What is the appropriate duration of treatment for uncomplicated cellulitis?

In patients with uncomplicated cellulitis, 5 days of antibiotics appears to be as effective as 10 days of therapy as long as there is initial and continued improvement.

This question was addressed in a single-center randomized controlled trial in which 121 patients aged ≥18 years with cellulitis of the face, trunk, or extremities were given 5 days of levofloxacin 500 mg PO daily and then randomized to receive either an additional 5 days of levofloxacin or placebo.[4] Exclusion criteria included bacteremia, severe sepsis, deep soft tissue infection (e.g., abscess, osteomyelitis, fasciitis), need for debridement, diabetic foot infection with nonviable tissue, bite, or eGFR <10 mL/min. After 5 days of levofloxacin, 34/121 patients were not randomized, including 6 who developed abscess, 1 who developed bacteremia, 4 who were worse by 72 hours, and 5 who did not demonstrate any improvement by 5 days. The primary outcome was resolution of the infection at 14 days as defined by cessation of warmth and tenderness, improvement in erythema, and no recurrence at the same site by day 28.

There was no difference in the primary outcome (98% in both groups; $P > .05$). Caveats include the fact that patients worsening before 5 days were removed and not randomized, which likely led to lower than average treatment failure rates in either group, as well as the choice of levofloxacin—a somewhat atypical agent for cellulitis treatment.

Based on this article, IDSA guidelines recommend a 5-day course of antibiotics for uncomplicated cellulitis, noting this can be prolonged in the absence of improvement during the course (strong recommendation, high evidence).[5]

---

[4]Hepburn ML, et al. Comparison of short-course (5 days) and standard (10 days) treatment for uncomplicated cellulitis. *Arch Intern Med*. 2004;164(15):1669-1674.
[5]See footnote 3.

Because he has no abscess or deeper/more severe infection, you inform the patient you plan for a short course of antibiotics, presuming he does not worsen at 72 hours and demonstrates some improvement by 5 days.

You are paged by the ED for an admission. A 63-year-old man with hypertension and hyperlipidemia presented with right forearm swelling and erythema. An ultrasound finds a 3.8 cm fluid collection concerning for abscess. He undergoes incision and drainage with purulent material expressed. He is feeling much better but develops chest pain during the drainage and is admitted to rule out myocardial infarction. You wonder whether he needs further antibiotics for his infection.

Do patients with skin abscess benefit from antibiotics beyond drainage?

Patients with skin abscess have higher cure rates when drainage is followed by 7 to 10 days of antibiotics.

A double blinded, placebo-controlled trial evaluated the effect of antibiotics on cure rates after skin abscess exploration among 1247 patients at five US EDs in MRSA-prevalent areas.[6] Patients ≥12 years old with abscesses ≥2 cm for <1 week were randomized after drainage to either TMP-SMX or placebo for 7 days. Exclusion criteria included suspected osteomyelitis or septic arthritis, diabetic foot infection, mammalian bite, intravenous drug use within the previous month along with fever, long-term care residence, immunodeficiency, and renal impairment.

The primary outcome was clinical cure, as defined by the absence of any failure criteria at each of three successive visits: fever, increase in erythema, worsening of swelling, and tenderness at day 3 to 4; fever, no decrease in erythema, swelling, tenderness at day 8 to 10; fever, more than minimal erythema, swelling, tenderness at day 14 to 21. Secondary outcomes included need for surgical drainage, recurrent infection, invasive infection, and hospitalization.

The primary outcome occurred in a greater proportion of the TMP-SMX than the placebo group (92.9% vs. 85.7%; $P < .001$). There was

[6]Talan DA, et al. Trimethoprim–sulfamethoxazole versus placebo for uncomplicated skin abscess. *N Engl J Med*. 2016;374(9):823-832.

no difference between the groups in recurrent infection or hospitalization. The authors reported a statistically significant reduction in the rate of additional surgical drainage in the TMP-SMX group (3.4% vs. 8.6%; *P*-value not reported). A caveat is that patients in this study had mostly small abscesses (median length 2.5 cm) with relatively significant surrounding erythema (median length 6.5 cm), potentially limiting applicability of findings to more prominent abscess without surrounding cellulitis.

A 2018 systematic review and meta-analysis[7] assessed 14 randomized clinical trials comparing antibiotics either to no antibiotics or other antibiotics among pediatric and adult patients with uncomplicated skin abscess. Antibiotics with MRSA activity (trimethoprim-sulfamethoxazole and clindamycin) were associated with lower rates of treatment failure than placebo (OR 0.45, 95% CI 0.33-0.62; no *P*-value reported). Conversely, antibiotics without MRSA activity (first-generation cephalosporins) did not demonstrate reductions in treatment failure compared to placebo (OR 1.82, 95% CI 0.68-4.85; no *P*-value reported). This meta-analysis is limited by variable patient populations and outcome definitions in component studies, as well as changing microbiology and resistance patterns between studies conducted decades apart.

After considering local antibiotic resistance patterns, treatment side effects, and patient preferences, you prescribe a course of TMP-SMX following drainage of his abscess.

A 68-year-old woman with hypertension, hyperlipidemia, coronary artery disease, and type 2 diabetes complicated by neuropathy presents to the ED with chills, right foot pain, and erythema extending over the right foot and up the ankle. On examination, she is found to have a 2 cm by 1 cm ulceration on the plantar surface of her foot that probes to bone. Her labs are notable for WBC 16 K/µL, CRP 110 mg/L, and ESR 80 mm/h. X-ray of her foot shows soft tissue swelling, but no gas or periosteal changes. You suspect osteomyelitis.

[7]Wang W, et al. Antibiotics for uncomplicated skin abscesses: systematic review and network meta-analysis. *BMJ Open*. 2018;8:e020991.

In diabetic patients with lower extremity ulcers, which signs and laboratory findings are most helpful in ruling in or out osteomyelitis?

In diabetic patients with lower extremity ulcers, an ulcer area >2 cm², probing to bone on examination, and erythrocyte sedimentation rate (ESR) >70 mm/h are very helpful to rule in osteomyelitis. The absence of these findings is only mildly helpful in ruling out osteomyelitis.

This question was addressed in a meta-analysis of 21 studies of 1027 diabetic patients with lower extremity ulcers.[8] Studies were included if data on history, physical, or laboratory values were extractable and compared to bone biopsy. Several features were particularly useful for ruling in osteomyelitis, including ESR >70 mm/h (+LR [likelihood ratio] 11, 95% CI 1.6-79), ulcer area >2 cm² (+LR 7.2, 95%CI 1.1-49), and positive probe-to-bone test (+LR 6.4, 95% CI 3.6-11). In terms of ruling out osteomyelitis, these tests are only somewhat useful, with ESR <70 mm/hr (−LR 0.34, 95% CI 0.06-1.9), negative probe-to-bone (−LR 0.39, 95% CI 0.2-0.76), and ulcer area <2 cm² (0.48, 95% CI 0.31-0.76).

Study caveats include variable quality of component studies with retrospective or unblinded designs, and the lack of assessment of diagnostic utility of combinations of variables. IDSA guidelines on diabetic foot infections[9] recommend probe-to-bone testing (strong, moderate) as part of the diagnostic workup for osteomyelitis in these patients.

You admit the patient with a high degree of suspicion for osteomyelitis. Your assessment is confirmed by bone biopsy.

A 58-year-old woman with multiple episodes of lower extremity cellulitis (including three hospitalizations in the last year) is admitted to your service with another episode of leg cellulitis, presumably secondary to streptococcus. You start her on IV antibiotics and admit her to the hospital. Over the course of 2 days she significantly improves. She is thankful for your care but frustrated that despite extensive outpatient efforts to identify and mitigate any potential predisposing factors (such as antifungal treatment of tinea pedis and compression stockings or diuretics for edema) she continues to have recurrent disease. She asks if there is any medication she can take to prevent future infections.

[8]Butalia S, et al. Does this patient with diabetes have osteomyelitis of the lower extremity? *J Am Med Assoc.* 2008;299(7):806-813.

[9]Lipsky BA, et al. Infectious Diseases Society of America clinical practice guideline for the diagnosis and treatment of diabetic foot infections. *Clin Infect Dis.* 2012;54(12):e132-e173.

What is the role of prophylactic antibiotics in patients with recurrent lower extremity cellulitis?

In patients with recurrent lower extremity cellulitis, prophylactic penicillin can decrease future infections.

In a multicenter, double blinded, placebo controlled randomized trial, 274 British patients with recurrent cellulitis were randomized to low-dose penicillin (250 mg PO BID) or placebo for 12 months.[10] Patients were included if they were ≥16 years old with recurrent cellulitis (≥2 episodes in the last 3 years, including ≥1 in the last 24 months). Exclusion criteria included existing antibiotic prophylaxis, previous surgery at the site, prior ulceration, or penetrating trauma. Patients were evaluated for recurrent episodes during the year of therapy (the prophylaxis phase) and the 2 years following (the follow-up phase). The primary outcome was time from randomization to first episode of recurrent cellulitis. Secondary outcomes included proportions with recurrent cellulitis during the prophylaxis and follow-up phases, and adverse drug events (including nausea, renal failure, diarrhea, and death).

During the prophylaxis phase there was a 45% reduction in the rate of cellulitis in the treatment group versus the placebo group (HR 0.55, 95% CI 0.35-0.86; $P = .01$; NNT = 5). After the year of prophylaxis, the rates of cellulitis in the follow-up phase were not significantly different (HR 1.08, 95% CI 0.61-1.98; $P = .78$). There was no significant difference in the number of participants reporting adverse events ($P = .5$) while taking prophylaxis. Caveats include small sample size, homogeneity of the population, and the lack of a formalized protocol for treating precipitating conditions.

A Cochrane review[11] of six trials (including the above study) encompassing 573 total patients further supports these findings, noting prophylaxis appears to be effective while it is taken but not after cessation. IDSA guidelines recommend consideration of prophylactic antibiotics for those with frequent cellulitis if efforts to treat predisposing factors are unsuccessful (weak recommendation, moderate evidence).[12]

> You provide the patient with a script for low-dose penicillin to start after completing the current course of antibiotics.

---

[10]Thomas KS, et al. Penicillin to prevent recurrent leg cellulitis. *N Engl J Med.* 2013;368(18):1695-1703.
[11]Dalal A, et al. Interventions for the prevention of recurrent erysipelas and cellulitis (review). *Cochrane Database Syst Rev.* 2017;6:CD009758.
[12]See footnote 3.

KEY LEARNING POINTS

1. In patients with cellulitis without abscess, empiric MRSA coverage does not significantly increase clinical cure rates as compared with empiric *Streptococcus* coverage alone.
2. In patients with uncomplicated cellulitis, 5 days of antibiotics appears to be as effective as 10 days of therapy as long as there is initial and continued improvement.
3. Patients with skin abscess have higher cure rates when drainage is followed by 7 to 10 days of antibiotics.
4. In diabetic patients with lower extremity ulcers, an ulcer area >2 cm^2, probing to bone on examination, and ESR >70 mm/h are very helpful to rule in osteomyelitis. The absence of these findings is only mildly helpful in ruling out osteomyelitis.
5. In patients with recurrent lower extremity cellulitis, prophylactic penicillin can decrease future infections, though infectious risk probably recurs after cessation of antibiotics.

ALCOHOL WITHDRAWAL

Rahul Ganatra, MD, MPH,
Scott Navarett, MD

You have just admitted a 63-year-old man with a history of coronary artery disease, diabetes, and alcohol use disorder for acute pancreatitis. He was previously drinking a "handle" (1.75 L) of vodka daily, but due to his current abdominal pain, has not consumed any alcohol in the past 72 hours. Review of the chart reveals multiple prior hospitalizations for alcohol withdrawal, including one requiring ICU admission. Since his arrival to the floor, the patient has received multiple doses of diazepam totaling approximately 200 mg in the last 24 hours, but remains tremulous and diaphoretic, and you worry his alcohol withdrawal could worsen significantly.

What features of a patient's history and current clinical presentation predict development of severe withdrawal?

Higher reported maximum 24-hour alcohol intake and number of prior withdrawal episodes are associated with severe withdrawal syndromes such as delirium tremens (DT) and/or seizures.

In a 1995 case-control study,[1] investigators used a large database of 1648 patients with DSM-III-R alcohol dependence enrolled at six academic medical centers across the United States to identify predictors of severe withdrawal. Among them, 12.8% (160 men, 51 women) reported the primary outcome of having had at least one episode of DT and/or seizures during an episode of withdrawal in the past.

---

[1]Schuckit MA, et al. The histories of withdrawal convulsions and delirium tremens in 1648 alcohol dependent subjects. *Addiction.* 1995;90(10):1335-1347.

Compared with alcohol-dependent patients who had never experienced an episode of DT and/or seizures, patients who had experienced these outcomes reported a higher number of drinks in any 24-hour period (OR = 1.02 per each additional drink, 95% CI 1.01-1.03; $P < .001$). Patients who had ever experienced an episode of DT and/or seizures also reported a higher number of antecedent withdrawal episodes (OR = 1.01 per each additional withdrawal episode, 95% CI 1.00-1.02; $P < .01$). Patients with a history of DT and/or seizures also reported more concomitant abuse of other sedative-hypnotic drugs ($P < .05$) and more chronic medical problems related to alcohol use ($P < .001$) compared with patients without a history of DT and/or seizures. Caveats in the interpretation of this study include its case-control design and reliance on self-report of both the exposures and outcome.

You recognize several high-risk features in his presentation, including his multiple prior episodes of withdrawal, high daily alcohol intake, and chronic medical problems. As you prepare to sign out, you inform the covering nocturnist that the patient is at high risk for complications of alcohol withdrawal. Overnight, the patient's condition worsens, and he requires transfer to the ICU for DT.

The following day, another new patient on your service, a 45-year-old woman with lower extremity cellulitis and a history of alcohol use disorder begins to develop signs and symptoms of alcohol withdrawal syndrome. Based on his experience caring for your previous patient who was sent to the ICU, the nurse asks if starting a scheduled benzodiazepine might be better for this patient than a symptom-triggered approach.

How does a fixed-dose approach compare with a symptom-triggered approach in treating alcohol withdrawal syndrome?

Administration of benzodiazepines via a symptom-triggered approach is the preferred treatment strategy over scheduled benzodiazepines for most patients because it leads to lower cumulative benzodiazepine doses and shorter hospital stays.

In a 1994 double-blind randomized controlled trial,[2] 101 patients admitted to an inpatient detoxification facility received chlordiazepoxide either on a fixed-dose schedule or as needed, based on a symptom-triggered administration schedule (the Clinical Institute Withdrawal Assessment for Alcohol, revised, or CIWA-Ar). Patients meeting DSM-III-R criteria for alcohol abuse or dependence admitted to a single Veterans Affairs Alcohol Detoxification Unit for management of acute withdrawal were included in the trial. Patients were excluded if they had any history of seizures or if they were already taking medications that could affect the clinical course of withdrawal, including opiates, benzodiazepines, barbiturates, clonidine, or β-blockers. All patients were reassessed by CIWA-Ar at baseline, every 8 hours, and every hour after benzodiazepines were administered. The primary outcomes were the duration of treatment and the total cumulative dose of benzodiazepines administered. Secondary outcomes included severity of withdrawal as measured by the CIWA-Ar score; against medical advice (AMA) discharges; development of hallucinosis, seizures, or DT; degree of general discomfort and alcohol craving; and rates of readmission and compliance with follow-up.

Treatment by a symptom-triggered approach was associated with a shorter duration of treatment (median 9 vs. 68 hours; $P < .001$) and a lower cumulative benzodiazepine dose (100 vs. 425 mg chlordiazepoxide; $P < .001$). There were no differences between groups in withdrawal severity, AMA discharges, episodes of seizures, or the development of DT.

Caveats in the interpretation of this study include the exclusion of patients with a prior history of seizures (this population may be at greater risk for developing complications from alcohol withdrawal) and that it was not powered to detect differences in secondary outcomes. Additionally, it is important to note that patients in the symptom-triggered group were reassessed by CIWA-Ar every hour after receiving a benzodiazepine. The net result of this frequent reassessment is that patients in the symptom-triggered group were dosed heavily up-front, effectively providing a loading dose early on in the course of their withdrawal syndrome.

---

[2]Saitz R, et al. Individualized treatment for alcohol withdrawal. A randomized double-blind controlled trial. *J Am Med Assoc.* 1994;272(7):519-523.

These results have been replicated in other inpatient alcohol detoxification populations, including patients with a history of seizures or DT.[3] Moreover, similar results have been demonstrated in subsequent observational studies in medical inpatients,[4] critically ill patients,[5] and ED patients.[6]

> You treat the patient with symptom-triggered diazepam. Three days later, she has fully recovered from both her cellulitis and alcohol withdrawal. The patient is hoping to use this moment of sobriety as an opportunity to finally quit alcohol for good, but is concerned that she may resume drinking once she returns home. You want to offer her the best chance at maintaining continued abstinence and wonder if any medications can help her do so.

What medications should be considered to reduce the risk of relapse in alcohol use disorder?

Acamprosate, oral naltrexone, intramuscular naltrexone, and disulfiram are U.S. Food and Drug Administration (FDA)-approved options for the treatment of alcohol use disorder.

Of the approved agents, strong clinical trial evidence supports the use of naltrexone. The largest of these trials was the COMBINE study, a randomized clinical trial of 1383 patients at 11 US academic centers. Patients were randomized to one of nine study arms, each of which included at least a minimum level of alcohol cessation counseling.[7] Patients in study arms 1 to 4 received medical management (placebo, acamprosate, naltrexone, or acamprosate + naltrexone); patients in arms 5 to 8 received the same medications plus enhanced alcohol cessation counseling, and patients in the ninth study arm received the enhanced

---

[3]Daeppen JB, et al. Symptom-triggered vs fixed-schedule doses of benzodiazepine for alcohol withdrawal: a randomized treatment trial. *Arch Intern Med*. 2002;162(10):1117-1121.
[4]Jaeger TM, Lohr RH, Pankratz VS. Symptom-triggered therapy for alcohol withdrawal syndrome in medical inpatients. *Mayo Clin Proc*. 2001;76(7):695-701.
[5]Decarolis DD, et al. Symptom-driven lorazepam protocol for treatment of severe alcohol withdrawal delirium in the intensive care unit. *Pharmacotherapy*. 2007;27(4):510-518.
[6]Cassidy EM, et al. Symptom-triggered benzodiazepine therapy for alcohol withdrawal syndrome in the emergency department: a comparison with the standard fixed dose benzodiazepine regimen. *Emerg Med J*. 2012;29(10):802-804.
[7]Anton RF, et al. Combined pharmacotherapies and behavioral interventions for alcohol dependence: the COMBINE study: a randomized controlled trial. *J Am Med Assoc*. 2006; 295(17):2003-2017.

alcohol cessation counseling alone. The authors performed a factorial analysis using patients in study arms 1 to 8. All patients received treatment for 16 weeks and were followed for up to 1 year. Primary outcomes were percent days abstinent from alcohol and time to first heavy drinking day (defined as ≥5 drinks for men, ≥4 for women).

Compared with patients receiving placebo and standard counseling alone, patients receiving naltrexone and standard counseling had a higher percentage of total days abstinent (80.6% vs. 75.1%; $P < .05$) and a reduced risk of a heavy drinking day (HR 0.72, 95% CI 0.53-0.98; $P = .02$). In general, groups who received naltrexone, enhanced counseling, or both, had the highest percentage of total days abstinent and the lowest risk of a heavy drinking day. Acamprosate, either alone or in combination with intensive counseling, was not associated with improvements in either total days abstinent or risk of a heavy drinking day compared with standard counseling alone.

Other studies, summarized in a 2010 Cochrane review,[8] have indicated more favorable outcomes with acamprosate than were observed in COMBINE. Included studies were randomized controlled trials that enrolled adults aged ≥18 years with alcohol dependence, were double-blinded, and compared acamprosate (alone or combined with other therapies) to placebo or an active control (including other pharmacotherapy). Twenty-four trials (including the COMBINE study) involving a total of 6915 patients were included. The primary outcomes were relapse of any drinking and duration of abstinence. Compared with placebo, acamprosate was associated with a reduced risk of any drinking (RR 0.86, 95% CI 0.81-0.91; $P < .001$) and an increase in the cumulative duration of abstinence by an average of 10.94 days (95% CI 5.08-16.81; $P < .001$).

Regarding disulfiram, a 1986 randomized trial in 605 US veterans[9] did not demonstrate an association between disulfiram and abstinence or time to first drink. However, authors demonstrated improvements in total number of drinking days among a subgroup that completed all assessment interviews, suggesting a benefit for the most highly motivated patients. This study is limited by its extensive exclusion criteria, resource-intensive follow-up approach (which likely improves uptake of a medication that requires patient cooperation and motivation for its effectiveness), and conclusions based on secondary outcomes in subgroups.

---

[8]Rosner S, et al. Acamprosate for alcohol dependence. *Cochrane Database Syst Rev.* 2010;(9):CD004332.

[9]Fuller RK, et al. Disulfiram treatment of alcoholism: a veterans administration cooperative study. *J Am Med Assoc.* 1986;256(11):1449-1455.

The National Institute on Alcohol Abuse and Alcoholism provides recommendations on the use of these agents in motivated patients to reduce risk of relapse. Based on consistent, high-quality patient-oriented evidence from multiple trials, acamprosate and naltrexone each carry an "A" recommendation, whereas on the basis of inconsistent, conflicting, and lower quality data, disulfiram carries a "B" recommendation.[10]

> You consult with an addiction medicine specialist and the patient's primary care physician, working closely with the patient to take an individualized approach. After considering the patient's preferences, personal and medical circumstances, and outpatient follow-up plans, as a team you decide to start her on intramuscular naltrexone.

KEY LEARNING POINTS

1. Higher reported maximum 24-hour alcohol intake and number of prior withdrawal episodes are associated with severe withdrawal syndromes such as DT and/or seizures.
2. Administration of benzodiazepines via a symptom-triggered approach is the preferred treatment strategy over scheduled benzodiazepines for most patients because it leads to lower cumulative benzodiazepine doses and shorter hospital stays.
3. Acamprosate, oral naltrexone, intramuscular naltrexone, and disulfiram are FDA-approved options for the treatment of alcohol use disorder.

[10]Arias AJ, Kranzler HR. Treatment of co-occurring alcohol and other drug use disorders. *Alcohol Res Health.* 2008;31(2):155-167.

CHAPTER 5

URINARY TRACT INFECTION

Maria Nardell, MD,
Jonathan Bortinger, MD

A 62-year-old woman with a history of multiple sclerosis and neu-rogenic bladder with urethral catheter was admitted overnight with lethargy. Before meeting the patient in the morning, you see that the urinalysis is positive for nitrites and pyuria. Her nurse asks you if you would like to begin treatment for a catheter-associated urinary tract infection (CAUTI).

Can a positive urinalysis provide sufficient evidence to diagnose CAUTI in a patient with an indwelling catheter?

In the absence of clinical correlation, a positive urinalysis does not nec-essarily predict a positive urine culture, and in turn a positive urine cul-ture is inadequate to diagnose CAUTI.

A prospective observational study in an urban New York public teaching hospital[1] assessed whether positive urinalysis could predict positive urine cultures in intensive care unit patients with indwelling catheters. For 4 months, in order to compare urinalysis and subsequent quantitative culture results, investigators collected urine samples from 106 randomly selected ICU patients with urethral catheters in place for >12 hours. Patients with genitourinary trauma or instrumentation prior to admission, urinary tract infection (UTI) diagnosed prior to admission, or anuria with urine production <15 mL/day were excluded.

---

[1]Schwartz D, Barone J. Correlation of urinalysis and dipstick results with catheter-associated urinary tract infections in surgical ICU patients. *Intensive Care Med.* 2006;32(11):1797-1801.

Positive urine cultures were defined as $\geq 10^5$ organisms/mL urine with ≤ 2 species present. The authors found 44 positive cultures out of 300 samples. Test characteristics for urinalysis findings were as follows:

Urinalysis finding	Sensitivity (95% CI)	Specificity (95% CI)	+LR (95% CI)	−LR (95% CI)
Nitrites	29.5% (17-45)	91.8% (88-95)	3.52 (2.3-5.3)	0.56 (0.6-0.9)
Leukocyte esterase	52% (36-67)	85% (80-89)	(2.0-6.7)	(0.4-0.8)
Nitrite + leukocyte esterase	20.5% (10-36)	95.7% (92-98)	4.76 (2.1-10.8)	0.83 (0.7-1.0)
WBC count >10	61% (46-75)	73% (67-78)	(1.7-3.1)	(0.4-0.8)
Urobilinogen ≤4.0	89% (75-96)	13% (9-18)	(0.9-1.2)	(0.4-2.1)
Yeast	15.9% (7-31)	92.6% (99-95)	(1.0-4.8)	(0.8-1.0)
Bacteria	64% (48-77)	67% (61-73)	(1.5-2.6)	(0.4-0.8)

Nitrites in urinalysis were 91.8% specific but only 29.5% sensitive for a positive culture, giving +LR (likelihood ratio) 3.52 (95% CI 2.3-5.3) and −LR 0.56 (95% CI 0.6-0.9). The most specific finding was the combination of nitrites and leukocyte esterase, which was 95.7% specific and 20.5% sensitive, with +LR 4.76 and −LR 0.83, respectively. This combination's only moderately diagnostic LRs, however, do not obviate the need for culture. An important study caveat is the high prevalence of candida and enterococci species without nitrite reductase activity, which may limit the applicability of findings about the utility of nitrites.

Another study[2] performed in Texas sought to determine whether bacteriuria identified based on positive urine cultures correlated with symptomatic episodes of CAUTI in patients with long-term urinary catheters over a year-long period. Patients were included if they were enrolled in a hospital-based home care program and had indwelling catheters for >14 days. No exclusion criteria were specified. Nurses collected urinary samples from 14 patients weekly for 5 to 6 weeks and then monthly

---

[2]Steward DK, et al. Failure of the urinalysis and quantitative urine culture in diagnosing symptomatic urinary tract infections in patients with long-term urinary catheters. *Am J Infect Control.* 1985;13(4):154-160.

thereafter. Outcomes included the number and colony counts of different bacterial species in specimens to assess the relationship of these findings to CAUTI incidence. Number and colony counts were also performed sequentially before, during, and after antibiotic courses. Clinical or microbiologic criteria for CAUTI were not clearly defined, and the diagnosis of CAUTI was instead at the discretion of attending physicians.

Results showed that 111/177 (63%) urine cultures grew $\geq 10^5$ cfu/mL of two to four different microbial species. Only three patients experienced fevers during the trial, each of which was diagnosed as CAUTI; one patient was diagnosed twice. In these patients, 3/4 urine cultures were sterilized during antibiotic treatment, but microorganisms returned to their same concentration 2 to 12 days after therapy, further supporting the idea that colonization is common and does not correlate with febrile episodes.

Study caveats included small size and failure to clearly delineate the symptoms defining a CAUTI nor the required workup to rule out other causes of incident fevers. Given that CAUTI symptoms are particularly challenging to interpret since typical UTI symptoms (e.g., dysuria, urgency) may be absent with an indwelling catheter in place, these issues limit the applicability of this study.

Nonetheless, this study supports the idea that without clinical correlation, urine cultures cannot diagnose CAUTIs given that indwelling catheters are commonly colonized with bacterial concentrations at levels consistent with CAUTI microbiologic criteria, with or without symptoms, and even soon after antibiotics. IDSA defines CAUTIs based on a microbiologic finding ($\geq 10^5$ cfu/mL of ≥ 1 bacterial species) in combination with compatible clinical criteria (either genitourinary signs and symptoms or nonspecific findings such as fever or altered mental status, after other causes have been excluded).[3]

You tell the patient's nurse that you would like to defer antibiotics at this time based on the positive urinalysis alone. However, upon examining the patient and discovering new reported flank pain, you suspect her urine culture may be positive and she may in fact have a CAUTI that merits empiric treatment. Her examination is otherwise nonfocal and a preliminary infectious workup is negative; you now strongly suspect a CAUTI. You wonder whether before starting these antibiotics you should exchange her long-standing urinary catheter.

[3]Hooton TM, et al. Diagnosis, prevention, and treatment of catheter associated urinary tract infection in adults: 2009 international clinical practice guidelines from the Infectious Diseases Society of America. *Clin Infect Dis.* 2010;50(5):625-663.

Should an indwelling urinary catheter be exchanged at the time of treatment for a suspected CAUTI?

An indwelling urinary catheter that has been present for >2 weeks should be exchanged before culturing urine and initiating antibiotics.

This question was addressed in a randomized trial that assessed the effect of catheter exchange prior to culture and initiation of antibiotics among 64 elderly patients with permanent indwelling catheters and CAUTI.[4] Patients were included if they were long-term residents of free-standing geriatric centers and had symptoms and signs consistent with UTI. Patients were randomized to either catheter exchange or nonexchange before antibiotic therapy. Both groups received empiric quinolone antibiotics until sensitivities were known. Catheters had last been replaced on average 31 days prior to trial entry. The majority of patients had fever and leukocytosis, and 25% had bacteremia. In the exchange group, urine cultures were obtained both before and after replacement. Both clinical and bacteriological outcomes were measured at multiple time points, up to 28 days after completion of antibiotic therapy. Clinical outcomes were based on trends in signs of infection (including cure or improvement), as well as either treatment failure (persistence) or recurrence (improvement followed by worsening). Bacteriological outcomes were based on bacteriuric clearance after antibiotics at various time points.

Patients in the exchange group were more likely to be cured or improved at 3 days (25 vs. 11; $P < .001$) and at 28 days after therapy (24 vs. 16; $P < .001$). Patients with exchanged catheters also had a lower mean number of days of fever (2.9 vs. 4.6 days; $P = .05$). Patients in the exchange group were more likely to have a negative repeat urine culture at day 3 (24 vs. 8, $P < .001$), 7 days after treatment completion (18 vs. 9; $P = .01$), and 28 days after treatment completion (13 vs. 5; $P = .02$). The authors hypothesized that exchanging urinary catheters led to decreases in biofilms with resultant bacterial and clinical improvement. Limitations of this study include size and multiple outcomes.

The reduction in bacterial and biofilm burden after catheter change is further supported by a cross-sectional study[5] of 62 women ≥60 years

---

[4]Raz R, Schiller D, Nicolle LE. Chronic indwelling catheter replacement before antimicrobial therapy for symptomatic urinary tract infection. *J Urol.* 2000;164(4):1254-1258.

[5]Tenney JH, Warren JW. Bacteriuria in women with long-term catheters: paired comparison of indwelling and replacement catheters. *J Infect Dis.* 1988;157(1):199-202.

of age with chronic indwelling catheters and without UTI symptoms or current antibiotics. Compared to cultures from a long-standing catheter, urine cultured immediately after catheter change had both lower mean bacterial concentrations ($10^{6.4}$ vs. $10^{7.6}$ cfu/mL; $P < .001$) and fewer distinct organisms (2.5 vs. 4.0; $P < .001$).

Based on these results, IDSA guidelines recommend that in the setting of suspected CAUTI, indwelling catheters present for >2 weeks be replaced (A-I) and that cultures be drawn from the new catheter prior to administration of antibiotics (A-II).[6]

> You ask the nurse to replace the patient's catheter before obtaining a urine culture and initiating empiric antibiotics. The urine culture returns positive with a susceptible pathogen, and antibiotics are further narrowed. The patient's symptoms improve, and she is ultimately able to return home.
>
> You continue to your next patient, a 72-year-old woman who is admitted with a UTI for the third time this year. Her outpatient providers completed an extensive diagnostic evaluation which did not reveal an underlying cause of recurrent disease, and empiric trials of vaginal estrogen were unsuccessful. She asks if you can prescribe anything to reduce the frequency of her UTIs.

Should women with recurrent UTIs be prescribed prophylactic antibiotics to prevent future infections?

Prophylactic antibiotics are a reasonable option for postmenopausal women with recurrent UTIs but appear more effective in younger women.

A 2017 systematic review and meta-analysis of three randomized trials encompassing 534 postmenopausal women sought to answer questions related to long-term prophylactic antibiotic use to prevent UTIs in older adults.[7] The primary outcome was the rate of UTI recurrence during the prophylaxis period. UTIs were defined as $>10^5$ cfu/mL in urine culture and/or clinically (defined as dysuria, polyuria, flank pain, fever).

---

[6]See footnote 3.

[7]Ahmed H, et al. Long-term antibiotics for prevention of recurrent urinary tract infection in older adults: systematic review and meta-analysis of randomized trials. *BMJ Open.* 2017;7:e015233.

Inclusion criteria included English language randomized controlled trials comparing long-term antibiotic use (≥ 6 months) versus placebo or nonantibiotic use on the rate of UTI in older adults with a history of recurrent UTIs (≥ 2 in 6 months or ≥ 3 in 12 months). Older adults were defined as anyone ≥ 65 years or postmenopausal women of any age, though ultimately none of the included studies involved men. Studies were excluded if they focused on otherwise limited situations (such as postcatheterization, postsurgery, or in patients with spinal injuries or structural renal tract abnormalities). In each selected trial, intervention arms included 6 to 12 months of antibiotic prophylaxis (trimethoprim-sulfamethoxazole in one study and nitrofurantoin in the others). Control arms consisted of nonantibiotic prophylaxis (lactobacilli, vaginal estrogens, and D-mannose powder, respectively).

Random effects meta-analysis showed that during the prophylaxis period, women experience a lower risk of developing UTI (pooled RR 0.76, 95% CI 0.61-0.95; $P = .02$, NNT = 8.5), though one study suggested this benefit was lost 3 months after treatment. Adverse events varied across studies but included rash, gastrointestinal upset, and vaginal symptoms. The number of events requiring withdrawal from treatment was small in all studies. One study addressed antibiotic resistance and found it to be higher in women receiving trimethoprim-sulfamethoxazole than those taking lactobacilli. Review authors found limitations in design and reporting in the selected studies, reporting one at high risk for bias. All three studies were small with short follow-up.

Prior to this study, a 2004 Cochrane Database meta-analysis had assessed the benefit of prophylactic antibiotics in younger, healthy women.[8] Trials involved nonpregnant women >14 years old with ≥ 2 uncomplicated UTIs in the last year and were excluded if involving women with urological surgery, nephrolithiasis, or renal impairment. Ten of the included trials representing a total of 430 patients studied an antibiotic versus placebo, while the remaining compared different antibiotics. UTIs were defined both microbiologically (>10^5 bacteria/mL with bacterial identification or pyuria plus symptoms and >10^4 bacteria/mL) and clinically (dysuria or increased frequency). During the prophylaxis period, both microbial (RR 0.21, 95% CI 0.13-0.34; P-value not

---

[8]Albert X, et al. Antibiotics for preventing recurrent urinary tract infection in non-pregnant women. *Cochrane Database Syst Rev.* 2004;(3):CD001209.

reported; NNT = 1.85) and clinical (RR = 0.15, 95% CI 0.08-0.28, *P*-value not reported; NNT = 1.85) recurrences declined with antibiotic therapy.

Caveats for both of these studies include the lack of data on resultant antibiotic resistance and recurrence rates after the prophylaxis period.

After discussion and via shared decision making, you and the patient decide based on the potential for antibiotic resistance and concern about side effects to defer a prophylactic antibiotic regimen at this time.

KEY LEARNING POINTS

1. In the absence of clinical correlation, a positive urinalysis does not necessarily predict a positive urine culture, and in turn a positive urine culture is inadequate to diagnose CAUTI.
2. In the setting of suspected infection, long-standing (>2 weeks) urinary catheters should be exchanged prior to culture and antibiotics. These practices are associated with improvements in key clinical outcomes.
3. Prophylactic antibiotics may reduce the rate of recurrent UTIs in postmenopausal women, but appear to be more effective in younger women.

CHAPTER 6

SYNCOPE

Amrita Mukhopadhyay, MD,
Nicholas D. Patchett, MD

You are paged by orthopedic surgery about an elderly woman who was admitted to their service after an episode of unexplained syncope. The patient sustained an ulnar fracture during the fall, but the surgeon has decided that the fracture is nonoperative. The surgeon requests a consult about whether the patient's syncopal episode requires inpatient workup.

In the absence of other nonsyncopal conditions requiring hospital management, which patients with syncope can be safely discharged and which require hospital observation and workup?

Many patients with vasovagal, orthostatic, or medication-related syncope have outcomes similar to those without syncope and can therefore be safely discharged home. Patients with presentations concerning for cardiogenic syncope should be considered for admission.

A prospective cohort study[1] of 7814 participants in the Framingham Heart Study and the Framingham Offspring Study compared all-cause mortality among the 822 patients who experienced a syncopal episode during the study period, and 1644 age- and sex-matched control participants without a syncopal event. Mean age at enrollment was 51 and median follow-up was 17 years. For the 822 patients with a syncopal

---

[1]Soteriades ES, et al. Incidence and prognosis of syncope. *N Engl J Med*. 2002;347(12): 878-885.

episode, the cause was determined by physician panel consensus and categorized as *vasovagal, orthostatic, medication-related, cardiogenic, neurologic,* or *unknown etiology.* Outcomes assessed included all-cause mortality, myocardial infarction (MI) or death from coronary disease, and fatal or nonfatal stroke.

In multivariable analysis, patients with syncope from any cause had increased all-cause mortality (HR 1.31, 95% CI 1.14-1.51; $P < .001$) compared to those without syncope. However, when analyzed by etiologic subgroups, poor outcomes were primarily noted in patients with cardiogenic, and to a lesser extent, neurologic syncope. Compared to no syncope, cardiogenic syncope was associated with an increased risk of mortality (HR 2.01, 95% CI 1.48-2.73; $P < .001$), MI or death from coronary heart disease (HR 2.66, 95% CI 1.69-4.19; $P < .001$), and fatal or nonfatal stroke (HR 2.01, 95% CI 1.06-3.80; $P < .05$). Neurologic syncope was associated with increased mortality (HR 1.54, 95% CI 1.12-2.12; $P < .01$) as well as fatal and nonfatal stroke (HR 2.96, 95% CI 1.69-5.98; $P < .001$). On the other hand, the combined category of vasovagal, orthostatic, or medication-related syncope was not significantly associated with these outcomes.

A limitation of the study is that its outcomes are long-term, whereas the decision to admit a patient may be based primarily on preventing short- to medium-term harms. Other caveats include the observational design and racially homogeneous study population. The 2018 European Society of Cardiology syncope guidelines[2] make class I recommendations both against hospital-based evaluation for patients with reflex-mediated syncope in the absence of dangerous medical conditions, and for observation and potential admission for those with features suggestive of cardiogenic etiologies.

You evaluate the patient with a careful history, thorough physical examination, and an ECG. On your assessment, you find she has mild dementia that complicates efforts to elucidate key details. Therefore, you focus your interview on aspects of the history that can differentiate cardiogenic from the lower-risk etiologies of syncope.

---

[2]Brignole M, et al. 2018 ESC guidelines for the diagnosis and management of syncope. *Eur Heart J.* 2018;39(21):1883-1948.

What aspects of the patient-reported clinical history are most helpful for determining whether syncope is cardiogenic?

Syncope during effort, structural heart disease, and age ≥60 years can be very useful for differentiating between cardiogenic and noncardiogenic causes of syncope.

To derive a model of the most useful features of the history to predict cardiac syncope, a meta-analysis[3] used a derivation sample of seven studies representing a total of 2388 North American and European patients. Studies were included if they reported ≥2 historical features and their relationship to a final diagnosis of cardiac or noncardiac syncope. The strongest predictors of cardiac syncope were syncope during effort (LR 6.92; $P <$ .0001), supine syncope (LR 4.23; $P <$ .0001), structural heart disease (LR 3.00; $P <$ .0001), and age ≥60 years (LR not reported; $P <$ .0001). A caveat to these data is that component studies used variable definitions for syncope type and historical features. ACC/AHA/HRS guidelines[4] list exertional or supine syncope, structural heart disease, and age >60 years among the criteria predicting cardiac etiology.

You confirm that the patient is 78 years old. She tells you that she lost consciousness in a parking lot while walking from her car to the drug store. She is uncertain of the details of her medical history, and you will be unable to obtain her outpatient records over the weekend. However, she can tell you she was on her way to pick up refills of warfarin, which she takes for "irregular heartbeat," and also furosemide, which she takes "to keep fluid out of my legs."

Her age and syncope during effort make you concerned for a cardiac etiology, even prior to obtaining any formal workup. Most concerning is her presumed history of heart failure and atrial fibrillation, which may suggest underlying structural heart disease. You look at her ECG to see if it will further clarify her baseline cardiac pathology.

---

[3]Berecki-Gisolf J, et al. Identifying cardiac syncope based on clinical history: a literature-based model tested in four independent datasets. *PLoS One.* 2013;8(9):e75255.
[4]Shen WK, et al. 2017 ACC/AHA/HRS guideline for the evaluation and management of patients with syncope: a report of the American College of Cardiology/American Heart Association Task Force on Clinical Practice Guidelines, and the Heart Rhythm Society. *J Am Coll Cardiol.* 2017;136:e25-e59.

What ECG features are useful for stratifying syncope patients by mortality risk?

ECG findings shown to predict 1-year mortality in syncope patients include ventricular pacing, atrial fibrillation, left ventricular hypertrophy, and intraventricular conduction disturbances.

This question was addressed in a post-hoc analysis[5] of a prospective multicenter observational study of 524 patients in Spain presenting with syncope. Each had a readable ECG and 12 months of follow-up data. ECG findings associated with 1-year mortality on multivariate analysis were ventricular pacing (OR 21.8, 95% CI 4.1-115.3; $P < .001$), atrial fibrillation (OR 6.8, 95% CI 2.8-16.3; $P < .001$), left ventricular hypertrophy (OR 6.3, 95% CI 1.5-26.3; $P = .011$), and intraventricular conduction disturbances (OR 3.8, 95% CI 1.7-8.3; $P < .001$).

Limitations of this study include a low rate of subsequent sudden cardiac death (potentially due to high rates of subsequent pacemaker implantation among subjects), moderate sample sizes (limiting ability to make inferences about more rare ECG findings), as well as a single country design. The 2017 ACC/AHA/HRS syncope guidelines[6] include a class I recommendation to obtain an ECG for initial evaluation.

> The patient's ECG shows atrial fibrillation, nonspecific intraventricular conduction delay, and left ventricular hypertrophy. Given concern for underlying structural heart disease, you recommend that the patient stay the night for more workup. You consider whether you should also check orthostatic vital signs before admitting the patient.

How useful are orthostatic vital signs in evaluating syncope?

At least among older patients, orthostatic vital signs are a low-cost test that frequently changes management.

This question was addressed in a retrospective study of 2106 patients ≥65 years of age admitted with syncope. Authors assessed the costs associated with certain diagnostic tests and the frequency with which

---

[5]Pérez-Rodon J, et al. Prognostic value of the electrocardiogram in patients with syncope: data from the group for syncope study in the emergency room (GESINUR). *Heart Rhythm.* 2014;11(11):2035-2044.

[6]See footnote 4.

they changed management.[7] This study used two definitions of orthostatic hypotension: strict (drop in SBP ≥20 mm Hg, or a drop in DBP ≥10 mm Hg) and loose (SBP ≤90 mm Hg when standing). Other diagnostic tests evaluated in the study were: ECG, telemetry, transthoracic echocardiogram (TTE), cardiac enzymes, head imaging, electroencephalogram, and stress testing. Test reports, progress notes, and discharge summaries were examined using standard abstraction forms to determine whether results affected diagnosis, helped determine the etiology of syncope, and/or affected management. Estimated costs for each test were calculated using standard billing charges, nursing time, and wages.

Compared to all other diagnostic tests assessed, orthostatic vital signs changed management most frequently (25% of the time using the strict definition and 30% using the loose definition). All other tests affected management <13% of the time. Additionally, orthostatic vital signs were the least costly test, being estimated to cost only $5. Despite this, orthostatic vital signs were only conducted on 38% of admissions, compared to other common testing modalities, such as ECG, telemetry, and cardiac enzymes, each of which were performed on >95% of syncope admissions. Study caveats include the retrospective nature and single-centered design, the possibility that orthostatic patients could have another unrecognized etiology of syncope, as well as the challenges of assessing the impact of a negative diagnostic test on management. ACC/AHA/HRS[8] and ESC[9] guidelines each make Class I recommendations for orthostatic vital signs at initial evaluation.

> The patient's orthostatic vital signs are negative. You remain most concerned for a cardiac cause and consider ordering a TTE.

Which syncope patients should undergo TTE?

Patients with history, physical, or ECG suggestive of structural heart disease should have an echocardiogram to confirm or refute the suspected diagnosis.

---

[7]Mendu ML, et al. Yield of diagnostic tests in evaluating syncopal episodes in older patients. *Arch Intern Med.* 2009;169(14):1299-1305.

[8]See footnote 4.

[9]See footnote 2.

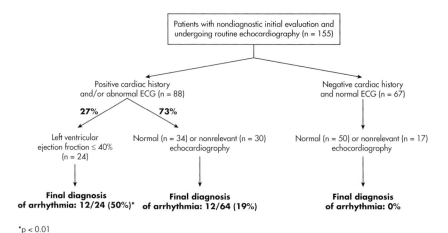

Figure 6.1 Diagnostic utility of TTE in patients with nondiagnostic initial evaluation. (From Sarasin FP et al. Role of echocardiography in the evaluation of syncope: a prospective study. *Heart*. 2002;88(4):363-367, used with permission from *BMJ Publishing Group Ltd.*)

A prospective observational study[10] of 650 patients at a single Swiss academic medical center aimed to characterize the diagnostic utility of TTE in syncope. Adult patients were included if they presented with a chief complaint of syncope. Syncope was characterized by strict diagnostic criteria into vasovagal, neurologic and psychiatric, orthostatic, carotid sinus hypersensitivity, and cardiac etiologies. All patients received a standard evaluation including history, physical (including orthostatic vital signs), labs, and ECG.

Following this standard evaluation, 155 patients (24% of the overall study population) had no proven or suspected etiology for their syncopal episode. These patients were separated into two groups based on the absence (67/155) or presence (88/155) of known or suspected underlying cardiac disease. Each received sequential cardiovascular testing starting with a TTE to assess for a cardiac cause of syncope and was followed for 18 months.

Among the 67 without suggestion of underlying heart disease by standard evaluation, TTE was either normal or demonstrated nonrelevant findings in all, and none were ultimately diagnosed with arrhythmia. However, among the 88 patients whose standard evaluation demonstrated known or suspected heart disease, 24 (27%) were found to have a left ventricular ejection fraction (LVEF) ≤ 40%. Half (12/24) of these

---

[10]Sarasin FP, et al. Role of echocardiography in the evaluation of syncope: a prospective study. *Heart*. 2002;88(4):363-367.

patients would ultimately be diagnosed with arrhythmia as the cause of their syncope (Figure 6.1).

The authors of this study suggest that TTE is useful to corroborate or characterize relevant structural cardiac abnormalities that are previously known or that are suspected based on standard evaluation. They also suggest that TTE is helpful for detecting reduced LVEF among patients whose cause of syncope remains unclear when standard evaluation is suggestive of underlying cardiac disease. Study limitations include its single-centered design and moderate sample size.

ACC/AHA/HRS[11] and ESC[12] guidelines recommend a TTE when there is suspicion of structural heart disease (Class IIa and Class I, respectively).

> The patient's echocardiogram reveals a left ventricular ejection fraction of 35% with inferior hypokinesis, findings the echocardiographer is able to confirm are old after accessing cardiology clinic records. The patient rules out for MI, but you are soon called to the bedside because she has experienced an episode of sustained ventricular tachycardia and recurrent syncope.

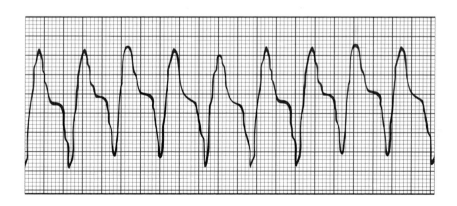

---

[11]See footnote 4.
[12]See footnote 2.

KEY LEARNING POINTS

1. Many patients with vasovagal, orthostatic, or medication-related syncope have outcomes similar to those without syncope and can therefore be safely discharged home. Patients with presentations concerning for cardiogenic syncope should be considered for admission.

2. Syncope during effort, structural heart disease, and age ≥60 years can be very useful for differentiating between cardiogenic and non-cardiogenic causes of syncope.

3. ECG findings shown to predict 1-year mortality in syncope patients include ventricular pacing, atrial fibrillation, left ventricular hypertrophy, and intraventricular conduction disturbances.

4. At least among older patients with syncope, orthostatic vital signs are a low-cost test that frequently changes management.

5. Syncope patients with history, physical, or ECG suggestive of structural heart disease should have an echocardiogram to confirm or refute the suspected diagnosis.

CHAPTER 7

STROKE

Jonathan Wang, MD,
Dawn Lei, MD,
Zahir Kanjee, MD, MPH

The ED physician calls you to admit a patient for symptom management related to a presumed diagnosis of peripheral vestibular neuritis. The patient is a 67-year-old man with a history of hypertension and hyperlipidemia who presented after 6 hours of new-onset intense vertigo, nausea, vomiting, and a feeling of postural instability. He reports a viral illness a week ago. You wonder whether this acute vestibular syndrome could in fact be caused by a posterior stroke, an important question given the potentially devastating and rapidly life-threatening nature of such a diagnosis.

What bedside testing can be performed to diagnose a posterior stroke in patients who present with the acute vestibular syndrome?

Head-Impulse-Nystagmus-Test-of-Skew (HINTS) testing can reliably assist in the identification of a posterior fossa stroke in patients presenting with acute vestibular syndrome.

In 2009, a prospective cross-sectional study addressed this question by evaluating 101 ED patients who presented with acute vestibular syndrome. [1] Subjects presented with a complaint of acute onset vertigo, nausea, vomiting, and unsteady gait. To be included, patients were required to have ≥1 stroke risk factor, such as hypertension, hyperlipidemia, atrial fibrillation, or prior stroke. Those with a history of recurrent vertigo or dizziness were

---

[1]Kattah JC, et al. HINTS to diagnose stroke in the acute vestibular syndrome: three-step bedside oculomotor examination more sensitive than early MRI diffusion-weighted imaging. *Stroke.* 2009;40(11):3504-3510.

excluded. Patients were clinically examined by a neuro-ophthalmologist and underwent MRI with diffusion-weighted imaging (DWI). Neuro-ophthalmologists were blinded to any MRI results available at the time of their examination. The gold standard of stroke diagnosis was neuroimaging results (in almost every case, MRI); patients with an initially negative MRI whose serial neurologic examination or clinical course were concerning for stroke underwent repeat imaging.

Authors identified a diagnostically useful battery of maneuvers, abbreviated as HINTS, including: normal horizontal Head Impulse test

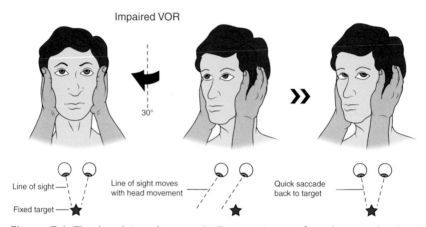

Figure 7.1 The head impulse test (HIT, sometimes referred to as the head thrust test) is a test of vestibular function that can be easily done during bedside examination. The HIT tests the vestibulo-ocular reflex (VOR) and can help to distinguish a peripheral process (vestibular neuritis) from a central one (cerebellar stroke). With the patient sitting on the stretcher, the physician instructs him to maintain his gaze on the examiner's nose. The physician holds the patient's head steady in the midline axis and then rapidly turns the head to about 20° off the midline. Panel 1: The normal response (intact VOR) is for the eyes to stay locked on the examiner's nose. Panel 2: The abnormal response (impaired VOR) is for the eyes to move with the head, and then to snap back in one corrective saccade to the examiner's nose. The HIT is usually "positive" (i.e., a corrective saccade is visible) with a peripheral lesion (vestibular neuritis), and the test is normal (no corrective saccade) in cerebellar stroke. This occurs because the VOR pathway does not loop through the cerebellum. Occasionally, patients with small brainstem strokes may have a positive test because the VOR pathway does loop through the brainstem. Because it is the "positive" test that is reassuring with the head impulse test and the "negative" test that is worrisome, it is very important to use the test only in patients with the acute vestibular syndrome (AVS). If one were to use the HIT in patients with pneumonia or with a fractured wrist, the HIT would be "negative" (worrisome for a central nervous system event). Therefore, it is critical that it only be applied to patients presenting with an AVS. (Reprinted from Wolfson AB, Cloutier RL, Hendey GW, Ling L, Rosen CL, Schaider J. *Harwood-Nuss Clinical Practice of Emergency Medicine.* Philadelphia: Wolters Kluwer; 2015, with permission.)

(Figure 7.1) (which indicates an intact vestibulo-ocular reflex—note: an abnormal reflex suggests a peripheral cause of vertigo); direction-changing Nystagmus with eccentric gaze; or Skew deviation (any vertical ocular misalignment, which may be best appreciated with covering/uncovering the eye).

The study found that the presence of any component of HINTS was 100% sensitive and 96% specific for a central lesion (73/76 of central lesions were posterior ischemic or hemorrhagic stroke), giving +LR (likelihood ratio) 25 (95% CI 3.66-170.59) and −LR 0.00 (95% CI 0.00-0.11). Indeed, the presence of skew deviation correctly identified an infarct in 7/8 cases where the initial MRI was falsely negative. Study authors highlight that the acronym INFARCT can be used to remember the danger signs of Impulse Normal, Fast-phase Alternating (referring to direction-changing nystagmus), Refixation on Cover Test (referring to skew deviation).

Notably, bedside testing in this study was conducted by a neuro-ophthalmologist, and use of these maneuvers by nonspecialists has not been adequately examined. Hospitalists should therefore be aware of the limitations of their nonspecialist HINTS examination in ruling in or out posterior stroke. The study was also limited to patients with acute, new-onset vertigo lasting hours and risk factors for stroke.

On HINTS testing, the patient exhibits a normal head impulse and abnormal cover test, both positive HINTS findings. This raises your concern for a posterior stroke and you order emergent MRI, which reveals a cerebellar infarction. The patient is admitted to the neuro ICU for management.

As you return to the medicine ward, you receive a stat page from a nurse who reports that one of your patients, a 63-year-old man with hypertension who is being treated for cellulitis, has just woken from sleep with acute aphasia and right-sided weakness concerning for a new stroke. He was last seen well when he went to bed about 9 hours ago. You see the patient and confirm the examination, finding him to have a moderate to severe stroke syndrome clinically consistent with ischemia in the left middle cerebral artery (MCA) territory, with National Institutes of Health stroke scale (NIHSS) of 16. His noncontrast head CT is unremarkable but a brain MRI shows a small infarct in the left MCA distribution. Given that he was last seen without deficits >6 hours ago, you know he is out of window for thrombolysis, but wonder if other directed therapies may be helpful.

Are any directed therapies beneficial in patients with acute stroke who were last seen well within 6 to 24 hours?

Mechanical thrombectomy can reduce disability in select stroke patients who were last seen well 6 to 24 hours ago when there is mismatch between deficit and infarct size.

The DAWN randomized clinical trial[2] assessed the impact of mechanical thrombectomy among 206 patients at 26 locations in North America, Europe, and Australia with a new stroke who were last seen well 6 to 24 hours prior. Adults ≥18 years old with occlusion of the intracranial internal carotid artery and/or the first segment of the MCA on CTA or MRA were included if they demonstrated a more severe neurologic deficit than would be expected based on their radiographic findings on CT perfusion or DWI MRI (suggesting a period when prompt reperfusion could prevent severe infarction). Patients were randomized to mechanical thrombectomy or usual care. Co-primary outcomes were level of disability (measured by utility-weighted modified Rankin scale, in which higher scores indicate decreasing disability) and rate of functional independence (measured by modified Rankin scale) assessed at 90 days. Secondary outcomes included safety and serious adverse events.

DAWN was stopped early for evidence of superiority. At 90 days, patients undergoing mechanical thrombectomy had lower disability (utility-weighted modified Rankin scale 5.5 vs. 3.4, posterior probability of superiority >0.999) and a higher rate of functional independence (49% vs. 13%, posterior probability of superiority >0.999). There were no differences in safety or serious adverse events. Caveats include the highly selected population with specialized comparisons of deficit and radiographic findings.

DAWN and the contemporary DEFUSE-3 study,[3] which found similarly impressive improvements in outcomes for thrombectomy in highly selected patients at 6 to 16 hours, led the AHA/ASA to issue strong recommendations for mechanical thrombectomy in selected stroke patients 6 to 24 hours after they were last seen well.[4]

[2]Nogueira RG, et al. Thrombectomy 6 to 24 hours after stroke with a mismatch between deficit and infarct. *N Engl J Med*. 2018;378(1):11-21.

[3]Albers GW, et al. Thrombectomy for stroke at 6 to 16 hours with selection by perfusion imaging. *N Engl J Med*. 2018;378(8):708-718.

[4]Powers WJ, et al. 2018 Guidelines for the early management of patients with acute ischemic stroke: a guideline for healthcare professionals from the American Heart Association/American Stroke Association. *Stroke*. 2018;49(3):e46-e110.

Neurology and radiology consultants discuss the MRI and conclude that the patient has a large mismatch between his severe clinical deficit and his mild MRI findings. As such, he undergoes mechanical thrombectomy. He does well with improvement in his deficits.

After an uneventful course in the neuro ICU for postprocedural observation, he is transferred back to your service. There is no obvious source of cardioembolism or other indication for anticoagulation. You want to start an antiplatelet agent, but the patient reports bronchospasm on previous exposure to aspirin.

What antiplatelet agent can be used in secondary prevention of noncardioembolic ischemic stroke in a patient with aspirin allergy or intolerance?

Clopidogrel monotherapy can be used in place of aspirin for secondary prevention of noncardioembolic ischemic stroke in patients who have an allergy or intolerance to aspirin.

This issue was evaluated in CAPRIE,[5] a randomized, multicenter, double-blinded trial across 16 countries of adults with atherosclerotic vascular disease such as recent (between 1 week and 6 months) ischemic stroke, recent (within 35 days) myocardial infarction (MI), or symptomatic peripheral arterial disease. A total of 19,185 patients were randomly assigned to clopidogrel 75 mg versus aspirin 325 mg daily and followed for 1 to 3 years. The primary outcome was the composite event rate of ischemic stroke, MI, or vascular death.

Patients receiving clopidogrel had a lower annual risk of the primary outcome (5.3% vs. 5.8%, RRR 8.7%, 95% CI 0.3-16.5; $P = .043$). Caveats to this study include the fact that the benefit for clopidogrel in the composite primary outcome appeared to be driven mostly by a subgroup with preexisting peripheral arterial disease rather than those with preexisting stroke. The trial's exclusion of stroke patients in the acute setting potentially limits generalizability to the initial poststroke period. Nonetheless, the evidence from CAPRIE was incorporated in the 2014 AHA/ASA guidelines recommending clopidogrel monotherapy as an acceptable choice for secondary prevention (Class IIa, Level of evidence B).[6]

---

[5]CAPRIE Steering Committee. A randomised, blinded, trial of clopidogrel versus aspirin in patients at risk of ischaemic events (CAPRIE). *Lancet.* 1996;348(9038):1329-1339.
[6]Kernan WN, et al. Guidelines for the prevention of stroke in patients with stroke and transient ischemic attack: a guideline for healthcare professionals from the American Heart Association/American Stroke Association. *Stroke.* 2014;45(7):2160-2236.

You start the patient on clopidogrel. Additionally, you recall that his home medication list includes low-dose simvastatin. You obtain a lipid profile that reveals a low-density lipoprotein cholesterol (LDL-C) level of 90 mg/dL.

What is the role of statin therapy in patients with prior ischemic stroke?

High-intensity statin therapy is recommended for secondary ischemic stroke prevention of presumed atherosclerotic origin, regardless of LDL-C level.

SPARCL[7] was a randomized, double-blind, multicenter clinical trial that randomized 4731 patients with recent stroke or transient ischemic attack (TIA), LDL-C level 100 to 190 mg/dL, and no known coronary heart disease to receive either atorvastatin 80 mg once daily or placebo. Patients were required to be discontinued off lipid-lowering agents ≥30 days prior to screening. The primary outcome was time to first stroke. Secondary outcomes included various cardiovascular and coronary events.

After adjusting for baseline differences, the primary outcome occurred at a lower rate in the atorvastatin group (HR 0.84, 95% CI 0.71-0.99; P = .03). Atorvastatin was associated with reductions in almost all secondary outcomes including major coronary event (P = .003) and major cardiovascular event (P = .002). The 2014 AHA/ASA guidelines recommend intensive statin therapy in ischemic stroke regardless of LDL-C levels (Class I; Level of evidence C).[8]

You initiate high-intensity atorvastatin therapy. Over several days, he recovers from his stroke symptoms and is ready for discharge. Standard inpatient evaluation, including brain imaging with MRI/MRA, vessel imaging with carotid duplex ultrasound, and cardiac evaluation with ECG, transthoracic echocardiogram, and telemetry monitoring, does not reveal a clear etiology for his ischemic stroke. You believe he has a cryptogenic stroke but know that the detection of atrial fibrillation would change your diagnosis and management. You wonder if a longer period of heart monitoring would be likely to demonstrate atrial fibrillation.

---

[7]Amarenco P, et al. High-dose atorvastatin after stroke or transient ischemic attack. *N Engl J Med.* 2006;355(6):549-559.
[8]See footnote 6.

How long should patients undergo heart rhythm monitoring for atrial fibrillation detection after suffering a cryptogenic stroke?

Cardiac monitoring for detection of occult atrial fibrillation is recommended for at least 30 days after an acute ischemic cryptogenic stroke or TIA.

The question about duration of cardiac rhythm monitoring for diagnosing atrial fibrillation in patients with cryptogenic stroke or TIA has been addressed in two randomized controlled trials. The first, EMBRACE,[9] enrolled 572 patients from 16 Canadian centers who were ≥55 years of age with cryptogenic ischemic stroke or TIA within the past 6 months and no prior history of atrial fibrillation. Cryptogenic stroke was diagnosed by a stroke neurologist after workup with brain and neurovascular imaging, 12-lead ECG, 24-hour ECG monitoring, and echocardiography. Participants were randomized to either conventional 24-hour ECG monitoring or 30 day event-triggered recorder. The primary outcome was ECG-documented atrial fibrillation lasting ≥30 seconds. Secondary outcomes included the proportion prescribed anticoagulation at 90 days. The event-triggered group had a higher rate of the primary outcome (16.1% vs. 3.2%; $P < .001$) and a higher proportion were prescribed anticoagulants at 90 days (18.6% vs. 11.1%; $P = .01$).

In the second study, CRYSTAL-AF,[10] the role of insertable cardiac monitoring (ICM) in detection of atrial fibrillation was evaluated among 441 patients from 55 centers across the North America and Europe who had suffered cryptogenic stroke or TIA within the past 90 days. Inclusion criteria included age ≥40 years and no prior history of atrial fibrillation. Patients were randomized to clinic follow-up and ECG monitoring at the site director's discretion versus an insertable loop cardiac monitor. The primary outcome was the rate of detection of atrial fibrillation >30 seconds at 6 months. Secondary outcomes included atrial fibrillation detection at 12 months, subsequent ischemic stroke or TIA, and anticoagulation use at 6 and 12 months.

---

[9]Gladstone DJ, et al. Atrial fibrillation in patients with cryptogenic stroke. *N Engl J Med.* 2014;370(26):2467-2477.
[10]Sanna T, et al. Cryptogenic stroke and underlying atrial fibrillation. *N Engl J Med.* 2014;370(26):2478-2486.

Compared to the control group, those with ICM had more detected atrial fibrillation at 6 months (8.9% vs. 1.4%, HR 6.4, 95% CI 1.9-21.7; $P < .001$) and 12 months (12.4% vs. 2.0%, HR 7.3, 95% CI 2.6-20.8; $P < .001$). At 12 months, more patients in the ICM group were on anticoagulation (14.7% vs. 6.0%, $P = .007$), but there was no difference in the rate of subsequent ischemic stroke or TIA (7.1% vs. 9.1%; P-value not reported).

Both EMBRACE and CRYSTAL-AF are limited by the fact that it is impossible to attribute the index event to a period of arrhythmia discovered afterward, that the periods of atrial fibrillation detected were relatively short, and that detection was not related to improvements in clinically meaningful outcomes such as recurrent stroke. Nonetheless, as a result of these trials, prolonged monitoring to detect occult atrial fibrillation is rapidly becoming standard of care after cryptogenic stroke or TIA.

> In your discharge planning with the patient and his primary care physician, you arrange for 30 days of outpatient cardiac monitoring to increase the possibility of diagnosing atrial fibrillation.

KEY LEARNING POINTS

1. HINTS testing can reliably assist in the identification of a posterior fossa stroke in patients presenting with acute vestibular syndrome.
2. Mechanical thrombectomy can reduce disability in select stroke patients who were last seen well 6 to 24 hours ago when there is mismatch between deficit and infarct size.
3. Clopidogrel monotherapy can be used in place of aspirin for secondary prevention of noncardioembolic ischemic stroke in patients who have an allergy or intolerance to aspirin.
4. High-intensity statin therapy is recommended for secondary ischemic stroke prevention of presumed atherosclerotic origin, regardless of LDL-C level.
5. Cardiac monitoring for detection of occult atrial fibrillation is recommended for at least 30 days after an acute ischemic cryptogenic stroke or TIA.

CHAPTER 8

GALLBLADDER DISEASE

Henry R. Kramer, MD,
Joseph S. Wallins, MD, MPH

A 40-year-old woman with hypertension and obesity presents to the ED with three episodes of upper abdominal pain and mild nausea of increasing severity and length over 2 weeks. On examination, she is afebrile and her vital signs are within normal limits. She has mild epigastric tenderness but is not jaundiced and has a negative Murphy's sign. Laboratory studies are unremarkable except for a left shift on her complete blood count with differential. She receives simethicone and viscous lidocaine, which partially improve her symptoms. You attribute her symptoms to mild gastritis and consider discharging her with primary care follow-up. However, you also weigh the potential diagnosis of acute cholecystitis and further imaging.

Are findings from a history and physical examination (H&P) sufficient for diagnosing or excluding acute cholecystitis?

Findings from the H&P alone are insufficient for diagnosing acute cholecystitis.

A 2017 systematic review and meta-analysis investigated the predictive power of various aspects of the diagnostic workup for acute cholecystitis.[1] The authors reviewed publications from 1965 to 2016 of patients presenting to the ED with a chief complaint of abdominal pain. Studies had to include findings of H&P, laboratory tests, or of ultrasound as well as a reference standard (either pathology or biliary

[1]Jain A, et al. History, physical examination, laboratory testing, and emergency department ultrasonography for the diagnosis of acute cholecystitis. *Acad Emerg Med.* 2017;24(3):281-297.

TABLE 8.1

Summary of Test Characteristics of Diagnostic Findings

Symptom/Sign	Sensitivity	Specificity	+LR	−LR
Fever	31%-62%	37%-74%	0.71-1.24	0.76-1.49
Jaundice	11%-14%	86%-99%	0.80-13.81	0.87-1.03
Right upper quadrant pain	56%-93%	0%-96%	0.92-14.02	0.46-7.86
Murphy's sign	53%-71%	95%-97%	11.48-21.31	0.32-0.50

scintigraphy). Three prospective observational studies with H&P information met inclusion criteria (Table 8.1). Among these, acute cholecystitis prevalence was 7% to 64%. Main outcomes included sensitivity, specificity, and LRs (likelihood ratios).

Lack of fever, jaundice, or Murphy's sign were not reliable to rule out acute cholecystitis, as the sensitivity of these signs was generally low. Notably, jaundice had very good specificity. The high specificity of Murphy's sign is tempered by the fact that it is based on a single study in which only 10.1% of the population had acute cholecystitis, and therefore false negatives were rare. Given small sample sizes and wide variations in acute cholecystitis prevalence, all of these studies are likely subject to selection bias. As a result, the diagnostic utility of several of these findings are likely overestimated.

EASL guidelines note that characteristic clinical signs and symptoms should raise a strong suspicion for acute cholecystitis but do not make recommendations for ruling out acute cholecystitis by H&P alone.[2]

You order a right upper quadrant ultrasound (RUQ US), which is reassuringly normal, and discharge her home with PCP follow-up.

The ED pages you for another admission, a 41-year-old woman with hypertension, hyperlipidemia, and obesity who presented with sharp right upper quadrant pain that began after eating a fatty meal. Her vital signs are stable. Laboratory studies, including transaminases

(continued)

[2]European Association for the Study of the Liver (EASL). EASL clinical practice guidelines on the prevention, diagnosis and treatment of gallstones. *J Hepatol.* 2016;65(1):146-181.

and lipase, are within normal limits. At the time of your evaluation about 2 hours after her arrival, she reports nearly complete resolution of symptoms. She notes her symptoms lasted about 3 hours and came in waves of pain. She reports one prior episode, which occurred several weeks earlier. You consider testing with a RUQ US to evaluate for cholelithiasis.

How accurate is RUQ US for diagnosing cholelithiasis?

RUQ US is adequately sensitive and very specific at diagnosing cholelithiasis.

This question was evaluated in a meta-analysis of the test characteristics of different imaging modalities for detecting cholelithiasis. Among articles published between 1966 and 1992, the authors included 30 studies with information on the sensitivity and specificity of various modalities.[3] Adjustments to sensitivities and specificities were made to account for verification bias (i.e., to account for systematic overestimation of sensitivity and underestimation of specificity arising from patients with positive RUQ US being more likely to undergo cholecystectomy, which was the most common gold standard for diagnosing gallstones). Ultrasound had an adjusted sensitivity of 84% (95% CI 76%-92%) and specificity of 99% (95% CI 97%-100%) for detecting cholelithiasis. According to the EASL, RUQ US is the initial imaging modality of choice for diagnosis of cholelithiasis (high quality evidence; strong recommendation).[4]

You order a RUQ US, which shows cholelithiasis without evidence of cholecystitis or choledocholithiasis. Aware that RUQ US can be of varying sensitivity for common bile duct (CBD) stones, you wonder whether the workup to date is adequate to rule out choledocholithiasis or if advanced diagnostics are necessary.

(continued)

---

[3]Shea JA, et al. Revised estimates of diagnostic test sensitivity and specificity in suspected biliary tract disease. *Arch Intern Med.* 1994;154(22):2573-2581.
[4]See footnote 2.

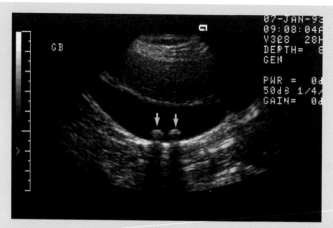

Reprinted from Willis MC. *Medical Terminology: The Language of Health Care.* Baltimore: Williams & Wilkins; 1996, with permission.

Which findings predict risk of choledocholithiasis?

Helpful predictive findings include the presence of cholecystitis, biliary pancreatitis, abnormal liver function tests, and CBD dilatation on ultrasound.

A prospective nonrandomized study at a single US academic center[5] assessed a risk stratification strategy for all patients undergoing cholecystectomy for cholelithiasis between January 1999 and April 2000.

Based on preoperative evaluation including H&P, lab tests, amylase, and RUQ US, patients were stratified into four groups of decreasing risk of choledocholithiasis. Risk criteria were based on previously performed research and included a pertinent clinical syndrome (cholecystitis, biliary pancreatitis, apparent resolving choledocholithiasis), abnormal liver function tests (≥ 2 of TBili ≥ 1.5 mg/dL, alkaline phosphatase >150 U/L, AST >100 U/L, or ALT >100 U/L), and CBD dilatation (≥ 5 mm) on RUQ US.

Patients with abnormal liver function tests and CBD dilatation without a pertinent clinical syndrome were assigned to group 1 and underwent ERCP (endoscopic retrograde cholangiopancreatography) prior to cholecystectomy with cholangiogram. Patients with a pertinent

[5]Liu TH, et al. Patient evaluation and management with selective use of magnetic resonance cholangiography and endoscopic retrograde cholangiopancreatography before laparoscopic cholecystectomy. *Ann Surg.* 2001;241(1):33-40.

clinical syndrome, CBD dilatation, and abnormal liver function tests were assigned to group 2 and underwent MRCP (magnetic resonance cholangiopancreatography) to assess for choledocholithiasis (in which case they underwent ERCP), followed by cholecystectomy and cholangiogram. Patients with a pertinent clinical syndrome and abnormal liver function tests without CBD dilatation were assigned to group 3 and underwent cholecystectomy and cholangiogram. Patients without a pertinent clinical syndrome, abnormal function tests, or CBD dilatation were assigned to group 4 and underwent cholecystectomy without cholangiogram.

Patients were followed for 30 days after surgery. The rate of choledocholithiasis in each group was a key outcome. Rates of choledocholithiasis varied across groups, ranging from 92.6% in group 1, 32.4% in group 2, 3.8% in group 3, and 0.9% in group 4 ($P < .001$). Caveats to this study include small sample size, single-centered design, the young age of the patients (which decreases external validity of CBD size criteria since dilatation increases with age), and the probability that diagnostic technologies have likely evolved in the intervening years since publication. Nonetheless, many of these criteria have been supported in subsequent studies. ASGE choledocholithiasis guidelines[6] recommend risk stratifying cholelithiasis patients based on several clinical predictors from this and other studies, including clinical syndrome, liver function tests, and CBD size on ultrasound, to determine whether to pursue advanced diagnostics before or with cholecystectomy.

Because she has NORMAL liver function tests and RUQ US does not show any CBD dilatation, you feel she is at low risk for choledocholithiasis and forego any advanced diagnostics for choledocholithiasis. You consider the optimal timing for cholecystectomy as definitive treatment for her biliary colic.

Should a patient with biliary colic be referred for early-interval cholecystectomy?

Referral for early-interval cholecystectomy after biliary colic reduces the risk of hospitalization or emergent cholecystectomy.

---

[6]American Society for Gastrointestinal Endoscopy Standards of Practice Committee. The role of endoscopy in the evaluation of suspected choledocholithiasis. *Gastro Endosc.* 2010;71(1):33-40.

This question was addressed in a 2016 retrospective study utilizing all Medicare claims data from 2001 to 2010 in Texas which assessed discharge follow-up,[7] a useful proxy for early-interval cholecystectomy. The authors included 11,126 patients ≥66 years presenting to the ED with symptomatic cholelithiasis and discharged home without immediate cholecystectomy or inpatient hospitalization. The care of these patients in the subsequent 2 years was assessed with follow-up care stratified as occurring with (1) a surgeon, (2) a nonsurgeon physician only, or (3) no physician follow-up. The outcomes of interest were the timing and rate of elective or emergent cholecystectomy or hospitalization for each patient stratum.

Most (76.8%) patients had follow-up with a surgeon and/or a non-surgeon physician. Patients following up with a surgeon underwent elective cholecystectomy the majority of the time (68.2%), with only 8.3% requiring emergent hospitalization or cholecystectomy. The rate of emergent hospitalization or cholecystectomy was nearly double for patients seeing a nonsurgeon physician only (14.6%). Patients without any physician follow-up fared the worst, with 77.6% requiring emergent hospitalization or cholecystectomy, the vast majority of which (95.9%) occurred within 2 weeks. Rates of emergent hospitalization or cholecystectomy differed across patient follow-up strata ($P < .0001$). Emergent cholecystectomy, compared with elective cholecystectomy, was associated with a higher perioperative mortality (3.8% vs. 0.9%; $P < .0001$) and a higher frequency of postprocedural complications (41.0% vs. 19.4%; $P < .0001$).

While the study does not directly address timing of surgery, the authors' conclusion—that timely outpatient surgical follow-up may help avoid emergent hospitalization and cholecystectomy—supports EASL guidelines, which recommend that uncomplicated biliary colic be treated with cholecystectomy as soon as possible (low quality evidence, weak recommendation).[8]

> You refer her for close surgical follow-up as an outpatient.

---

[7]Dimou FM, et al. Trends in follow-up of patients presenting to the emergency department with symptomatic cholelithiasis. *J Am Coll Surg.* 2016;222(4):377-384.
[8]See footnote 2.

KEY LEARNING POINTS

1. Findings from the H&P alone are insufficient for diagnosing acute cholecystitis.
2. RUQ US is adequately sensitive and very specific at diagnosing cholelithiasis.
3. Helpful predictive findings for choledocholithiasis include the presence of cholecystitis, biliary pancreatitis, abnormal liver function tests, and CBD dilatation on ultrasound.
4. Referral for early-interval cholecystectomy after biliary colic reduces the risk of hospitalization or emergent cholecystectomy.

MENINGITIS AND ENCEPHALITIS

Jennifer Hu, MD,
Amanda Cooke, MD

A 55-year-old man presents with fever, headache, photophobia, and altered mental status. On examination, he is febrile with mild nuchal rigidity. He is somnolent but arousable. You are concerned for meningitis or encephalitis and decide to proceed with lumbar puncture (LP). A colleague brings up the risk of herniation from LP and suggests delaying the procedure in order to obtain a head CT.

Which meningitis suspects require a head CT before LP?

Adults with a history of immunocompromise or central nervous system (CNS) disease (mass lesion, stroke, focal infection), new onset seizure, papilledema, abnormal level of consciousness, or focal neurologic deficit should undergo head CT prior to LP.

This question was addressed in a single-center prospective observational study at an urban academic ED of adults (>16 years) with clinically suspected meningitis.[1] Patients who had undergone CT scanning prior to enrollment or for alternate indications were excluded. The decision to undergo CT was at the discretion of the treating physician. Among patients who underwent CT, scans were categorized as normal (including isolated atrophy) or as having a focal (such as stroke or mass) or nonfocal (such as hemorrhage or hydrocephalus) abnormality. The presence and degree of mass effect was also noted in abnormal scans.

---

[1]Hasbun R, et al. Computed tomography of the head before lumbar puncture in adults with suspected meningitis. *N Engl J Med.* 2001;345(24):1727-1733.

Of 301 eligible patients, 235 (78%) underwent CT scan prior to LP, of whom 179 (76%) had normal CT scans and 56 (24%) had abnormal scans. Risk factors associated with abnormal CT include age >60 years ($P < .001$), immunocompromised state ($P = .01$), history of CNS disease ($P < .001$), seizure within 1 week prior to presentation ($P < .001$), reduced level of consciousness ($P < .001$), and abnormal focal neurologic signs on examination (such as gaze palsy [$P = .003$], visual field abnormality [$P < .001$], facial palsy [$P < .001$], arm/leg drift [$P < .001$], or abnormal language [$P < .001$]).

The above features were absent in 96 (41%) of the patients who underwent CT, with scans being normal in all but 3 of these 96 patients (NPV 97%). All three underwent LP without herniation. Four patients had mass effect on CT that led clinicians to defer LP, each of whom had at least one of the risk factors identified above.

Patients undergoing CT scan prior to LP had a delay in time from presentation to LP when compared to those who did not undergo CT (mean 5.3 vs. 3.0 hours; $P = .01$). Caveats include the study's single-centered setting and that head CTs were ordered at the discretion of the treating physician rather than routinely. Infectious Diseases Society of America (IDSA) guidelines recommend CT imaging prior to LP in patients with immunocompromised state, CNS disease, new onset seizure, papilledema, abnormal level of consciousness, or focal neurologic deficit (B-II).[2]

After an unremarkable head CT, you pursue LP. You order empiric antibiotics for meningitis and consider adjunctive treatment with dexamethasone.

Under what circumstances should patients with acute bacterial meningitis be treated with steroids?

Adults with suspected pneumococcal meningitis should receive early glucocorticoids before or at the time of antibiotic administration to reduce the risk of unfavorable outcomes including mortality.

This question was evaluated in a prospective, double-blinded, multicenter randomized control trial comparing early administration

---

[2]Tunkel AR, et al. Practice guidelines for bacterial meningitis. *Clin Infect Dis.* 2004;39(9): 1267-1284.

of adjunctive dexamethasone to placebo in 301 adults with suspected acute bacterial meningitis presenting to participating centers in the Netherlands, Germany, Austria, and Denmark.[3] Patients received either dexamethasone 10 mg (n = 157) or placebo (n = 144) 15 to 20 minutes prior to the first dose of antibiotics, which was continued every 6 hours for 4 days. This study included adults (age ≥17 years) with clinically suspected meningitis in combination with either cloudy cerebrospinal fluid (CSF), bacteria on CSF gram stain, or a CSF leukocyte count >1000/mm[3]. Patients with a CSF shunt or peptic ulcer disease were excluded. The primary outcome was the score on the Glasgow Outcome Scale (GOS), separated into "favorable" (mild or no disability) or "unfavorable" (ranging from moderate disability to death) categories. Secondary outcomes included mortality, focal neurologic abnormalities (defined as aphasia, cranial nerve palsy, monoparesis, hemiparesis, or severe ataxia), hearing loss, and clinically significant gastrointestinal bleeding. Prospective subgroup analyses were performed based on pathogenic organisms grouped as follows: *Neisseria meningitidis, Streptococcus pneumoniae*, other bacteria, or unidentified cause (negative CSF culture).

Compared to patients receiving placebo, patients treated with dexamethasone had lower mortality (7.0% vs. 14.6%, RR = 0.48, 95% CI 0.24-0.96; P = .04; NNT [number needed to treat] = 13.2) and fewer unfavorable GOS scores (14.6% vs. 25.0%, RR = 0.59, 95% CI 0.37-0.94; P = 0.03; NNT= 9.7). In subgroup analyses, the major differences in unfavorable GOS and mortality were noted in those with pneumococcal meningitis (P = .006 and P = .02, respectively). Dexamethasone did not significantly impact either of these outcomes for those with meningitis due to *N. meningitidis*, other bacteria, or unidentified cause. Dexamethasone did not affect rates of focal neurologic sequelae, hearing loss, or gastrointestinal bleeding.

In this study, the most frequently prescribed antibiotics were amoxicillin and penicillin, and all CSF samples submitted for analysis were susceptible to penicillin; however, this treatment regimen and resistance pattern is unusual in many areas of the world. Of note, trials of dexamethasone for bacterial meningitis in the developing world have demonstrated inconsistent results,[4,5] arguing that this study's findings may not be applicable in

---

[3]de Gans J, van de Beek D. Dexamethasone in adults with bacterial meningitis. *N Engl J Med*. 2002;347(20):1549-1556.

[4]Scarborough M, et al. Corticosteroids for bacterial meningitis in adults in sub-Saharan Africa. *N Engl J Med*. 2007;357(24):2441-2450.

[5]Nguyen TH, et al. Dexamethasone in Vietnamese adolescents and adults with bacterial meningitis. *N Engl J Med*. 2007;357(24):2431-2340.

all settings. Finally, because dexamethasone reduces blood-brain permeability and may impede penetration of vancomycin into the subarachnoid space, treatment failures have been reported in adults receiving adjunctive dexamethasone and standard doses of vancomycin.[6]

IDSA guidelines[7] make a strong recommendation for corticosteroids in suspected or proven pneumococcal meningitis (A-I) and suggest that steroids be offered in undifferentiated meningitis (B-III) until pneumococcus is ruled out. Experts also recommend that patients treated simultaneously with vancomycin and dexamethasone be closely monitored for treatment failure.

> The patient receives dexamethasone and antibiotics immediately after the LP. You know that postdural puncture headache (PDPH), a postural headache thought to be due to leakage of CSF through the hole in the dura created by the LP needle, is a possible complication of the procedure. The nurse asks if you are ordering postprocedural bedrest to prevent PDPH.

| Does postprocedural bedrest prevent PDPH?

Bedrest does not reduce the risk of PDPH.

In a 2016 meta-analysis, authors reviewed randomized controlled trials of activity restrictions (bedrest and/or head/body position) or fluid (oral or IV) to prevent PDPH.[8] These studies involved patients of all ages undergoing diagnostic or therapeutic LP. The primary outcome was the occurrence of PDPH (as defined by the International Headache Society or the individual studies) within 5 days of LP. Secondary outcomes included any headache after LP.

Meta-analysis of the 12 studies involving 1519 patients that compared bedrest to immediate mobilization found bedrest led to increased risk of PDPH (RR 1.24, 95% CI 1.04-1.48; P-value not reported) and any headache (RR 1.16, 95% CI 1.02-1.32; P-value not reported). Among the subset of six studies comprising 723 patients undergoing diagnostic LP, there was no significant difference between bedrest or

---

[6]Viladrich PF, et al. Evaluation of vancomycin for therapy of adult pneumococcal meningitis. *Antimicrob Agents Chemother.* 1991;35(12):2467-2472.

[7]See footnote 2.

[8]Arevalo-Rodriguez I, et al. Posture and fluids for preventing post-dural puncture headache. *Cochrane Database Syst Rev.* 2016;(3):CD009199.

immediate mobilization in the rate of PDPH (RR 1.11, 95% CI 0.90-1.37; *P*-value not reported) or any headache (RR 1.15, 95% CI 0.94-1.40; *P*-value not reported). Caveats include that some component studies were at high risk of bias due to lack of blinding.

> You allow him to ambulate in his room with assistance. Given your concern for encephalitis, you debate whether to empirically start acyclovir now or wait until herpes simplex virus (HSV) test results from the LP are available.

What are the risks of delaying acyclovir in HSV encephalitis?

Delay in empiric treatment is associated with unfavorable outcomes from HSV encephalitis.

To identify parameters independently associated with poor prognosis in HSV encephalitis, a 2002 multicenter retrospective case-control study of HSV encephalitis was conducted among adults treated with acyclovir.[9] Ninety-three patients with PCR-proven HSV-1 encephalitis from 36 French medical centers were included. Parameters retrieved from medical records included admission Glasgow Coma Scale, Simplified Acute Physiology Score (SAPS II), CSF profile, and timing and dose of acyclovir. The primary outcome was handicap and quality of life at 6 and 12 months, as graded according to a 5-point scale derived from the Glasgow Outcome Scale. Patients were categorized to have either a "favorable outcome" if they had complete recovery or mild to moderate disability or a "poor outcome" for those who died or suffered severe disability (requiring institutionalization or constant life aid).

Six months after the onset of HSV encephalitis, of the 85 patients who were not lost to follow-up, 13 (15%) had died and only 12 (14%) achieved complete recovery. In univariate analysis, patients who experienced poor outcome had significantly lower admission Glasgow Coma Scale scores. In multivariate analysis, two factors were associated with poor outcome: a delay of >2 days between admission and initiation of acyclovir therapy (OR 3.1, 95% CI 1.1-9.1; *P* = .037) and an elevated admission SAPS II (OR 3.7, 95% CI 1.3-10.6; *P* = .014). Patients with a

---

[9]Raschilas F, et al. Outcome of and prognostic factors for herpes simplex encephalitis in adult patients: results of a multicenter study. *Clin Infect Dis.* 2002;35(3):254-260.

favorable outcome had a shorter delay between admission and receipt of acyclovir, with 75% (n = 55) of those with a favorable outcome receiving acyclovir within 2 days of admission, as compared to 30% (n = 30) of those with a poor outcome ($P < .001$).

You promptly initiate the patient on acyclovir. His diagnosis is ultimately confirmed as pneumococcal meningitis and his regimen is narrowed appropriately. He improves and is eventually discharged to a rehabilitation facility.

KEY LEARNING POINTS

1. Adults with a history of immunocompromise or CNS disease (mass lesion, stroke, focal infection), new onset seizure, papilledema, abnormal level of consciousness, or focal neurologic deficit should undergo head CT prior to LP to rule out meningitis.
2. Adults with suspected pneumococcal meningitis should receive early glucocorticoids before or at the time of antibiotic administration to reduce the risk of unfavorable outcomes including mortality.
3. Bedrest does not reduce the risk of PDPH.
4. Delay in empiric treatment is associated with unfavorable outcomes from HSV encephalitis.

DIABETES AND HYPERGLYCEMIA

Anita Vanka, MD, FHM,
Celeste Pizza, MD

A 52-year-old woman with type 2 diabetes mellitus (DM) on metformin and glipizide is admitted to your service for right lower extremity cellulitis. Her oral antihyperglycemic agents are held on admission, and she is started on sliding scale insulin (SSI) lispro. Over the next 24 hours, you note her fingersticks are consistently between 195 to 220 mg/dL. Your resident advocates for starting a regimen to bring the patient's blood sugars down to 100 mg/dL in order to promote better healing from the cellulitis. You pose the following question to the team on rounds:

What are appropriate glycemic targets for hospitalized patients?

A glucose range of 140 to 180 mg/dL is recommended for the majority of patients.

NICE-SUGAR[1] was a multinational randomized controlled trial across 42 different hospitals in which 6104 medical and surgical ICU patients were randomized to intensive (goal 81-108 mg/dL) versus conventional (goal <180 mg/dL) glucose control approaches. Eligible patients were adults who were expected to require care in the ICU for ≥3 consecutive days. Exclusion criteria included admission to the ICU for diabetic ketoacidosis (DKA) or hyperosmolar state, or prior hypoglycemia without full neurological recovery. The primary outcome was

---

[1]NICE-SUGAR Study Investigators. Intensive versus conventional glucose control in critically ill patients. *N Engl J Med.* 2009;360(13):1283-1297.

death from any cause within 90 days. Secondary outcomes included hypoglycemia (≤40 mg/dL) as well as ICU and hospital length of stay.

The intensive control group had higher mortality (27.5% vs. 24.9% in the conventional control group, HR 1.11, 95% CI 1.01-1.23; $P = .03$) and more frequent hypoglycemia (6.8% vs. 0.5% in the conventional control group; $P < .001$). There were no differences between the groups in terms of ICU or overall hospital length of stay.

Based on the above study, the American Diabetes Association (ADA) recommends initiation of insulin for persistently elevated glucose levels ≥180 mg/dL with a target range of 140 to 180 mg/dL for the majority of critically and noncritically ill patients (grade A recommendation).[2]

> After discussing the NICE-SUGAR study results, your team establishes a glycemic target of 140 to 180 mg/dL for this patient. Your residents attempt to achieve this target using only SSI and a diabetic diet. However, over the next day, the patient's blood sugars continue to be above range. Your residents suggest increasing her SSI dose further to achieve glucose values <180 mg/dL. You ask them:

Should SSI be used as the sole form of insulin in hospitalized patients with type 2 DM?

Sole use of SSI is discouraged, as it results in higher blood sugars than basal-bolus insulin.

The RABBIT 2 trial[3] was a multicenter, randomized trial comparing basal-bolus insulin to SSI alone in type 2 diabetic patients. One hundred thirty insulin-naive type 2 diabetic patients without ketoacidosis were randomized to receive basal-bolus insulin with glargine plus glulisine insulin or SSI alone. Patients in the basal-bolus group were started on a weight-based regimen with scheduled glargine and glulisine insulin with an additional glulisine SSI. Patients in the SSI group received regular insulin four times daily if eating or every 6 hours if fasting for blood sugar >140 mg/dL. Patients in the ICU, on systemic corticosteroid

[2]American Diabetes Association. Standards of medical care in diabetes – 2019. *Diabetes Care.* 2019;42(suppl 1):S173-S181.

[3]Umpierrez GE, et al. Randomized study of basal-bolus insulin therapy in the inpatient management of patients with type 2 diabetes (RABBIT 2 trial). *Diabetes Care.* 2007;30(9):2181-2186.

therapy, or with known hepatic or renal disease (creatinine ≥3.0 mg/dL) were excluded. The primary outcome was mean daily blood glucose level. Secondary outcomes included frequency of hypoglycemia (<60 mg/dL), length of stay, and mortality.

Compared to those receiving basal-bolus, patients treated with SSI alone had higher mean daily (193 ± 54 vs. 166 ± 32 mg/dL; $P < .001$), fasting (165 ± 41 vs. 147 ± 36 mg/dL; $P < .01$), and random (189 ± 42 vs. 164 ± 35 mg/dL; $P < .001$) blood glucose levels. Compared to those in the basal-bolus group, fewer patients in the SSI group had mean glucose less than the 140 mg/dL target (38% vs. 66%; P-value not reported). Hypoglycemia occurred in two patients in each group (P-value not reported). Caveats of this trial include small sample size, limited treatment regimen options, and open-label protocol. ADA guidelines[4] recommend basal-bolus insulin for those with adequate nutrition (grade A recommendation) and advise against prolonged use of SSI alone (grade A recommendation).

> With basal-bolus insulin, she achieves euglycemia and is soon ready to be discharged home. Your team must now decide what to do with her home DM medications and whether to continue the insulin you started in the hospital. You note her recent hemoglobin A1C of 8.7%.

How can a recent hemoglobin A1C inform a discharge DM medication regimen?

Discharge medication algorithms based on hemoglobin A1C can lead to improved outpatient glycemic control.

Two prospective, multicenter open-label studies have assessed the safety and efficacy of hospital discharge algorithms based on admission hemoglobin A1C. In the most recent study,[5] patients who were already enrolled in the SITA-Hospital Trial (a multicenter randomized trial studying the effects of the addition of sitagliptin to inpatient insulin regimens) were invited to participate in a 6-month postdischarge study. Exclusion criteria included history of DKA, gastrointestinal obstruction,

---

[4]See footnote 2.
[5]Gianchandani RY, et al. The efficacy and safety of co-administration of sitagliptin with metformin in patients with type 2 diabetes at hospital discharge. *Endocr Pract.* 2018;24(6):556-564.

corticosteroid therapy, and glomerular filtration rate (GFR)<30 mL/min/1.73 m². A total of 253 medical and surgical patients agreed to participate and were grouped according to their hemoglobin A1C level as measured during the hospitalization. Patients with a hemoglobin A1C <7% (controlled group) were discharged on either sitagliptin and metformin (and, if they were on insulin prior to admission, 50% of their inpatient insulin dose) or resumed their previous preadmission diabetic regimen; those with a hemoglobin A1C 7% to 9% (moderately uncontrolled group) were discharged on sitagliptin and metformin plus insulin glargine at 50% of their hospital insulin dose; those with a hemoglobin A1C >9% (severely uncontrolled group) were discharged on sitagliptin and metformin plus insulin glargine at 80% of their hospital insulin dose. Patients all received education on home glucose monitoring and hypoglycemia. Patients self-monitored glucose and were followed up by telephone every 2 weeks and clinic visits 1, 3, and 6 months after discharge. Coprimary outcomes were change in hemoglobin A1C at 3 and 6 months post discharge. Secondary outcomes included hypoglycemia (glucose <70 mg/dL) and "clinically important hypoglycemia" (glucose <54 mg/dL).

Mean baseline hemoglobin A1C across all three groups was 8.7% ± 2.3%. This value decreased to 7.3% ± 1.5% (P < .001) at 3 months and 7.3% ± 1.7% at 6 months (P < .001). The moderately uncontrolled group had reductions in hemoglobin A1C from 8.0% to 7.3% at 3 and 6 months (P < .001 for each comparison to baseline), and the severely uncontrolled group had reductions in A1C from 11.3% to 8.0% at 3 and 6 months (P < .001 for each comparison to baseline). Glucose values < 70 mg/dL occurred in 23%, clinically important hypoglycemia occurred in 5%. Caveats of this study include the relatively intense follow-up which may not be realistic for all patients, the high cost of the study medication, small sample size, and observational nature.

The earlier study[6] was similar in that it included discharged patients who had been enrolled in a different inpatient randomized clinical trial (the Basal-Plus Trial, which studied the effects of inpatient insulin regimens). It followed 224 patients for 12 weeks post discharge with frequent telephone monitoring and occasional clinic visits. Groups were defined in the same way as in the trial above. The controlled group was

---

[6]Umpierrez GE, et al. Hospital discharge algorithm based on admission HbA1c for the management of patients with type 2 diabetes. *Diabetes Care*. 2014;37(11):2934-2939.

discharged on their preadmission regimen; the moderately uncontrolled group was discharged on preadmission oral agents plus insulin at 50% of their hospital daily dose; the severely uncontrolled group was discharged on preadmission oral agents plus insulin at 80% of their hospital daily dose.

Mean baseline hemoglobin A1C across the three groups was 8.5% ± 2.5% and decreased to 7.3% ± 1.5% at 12 weeks ($P < .001$). All three groups demonstrated a decrease in hemoglobin A1C at 12 weeks ($P < .001$ for each). The largest reduction was in the severely uncontrolled group, whose hemoglobin A1Cs decreased by 3.2% ± 2.4% compared to baseline ($P < .001$). Rates of glucose <70 mg/dL were 29%, with 3% having episodes of glucose <40 mg/dL. Limitations of this study include small sample size, intense follow-up, short follow-up interval, and a relatively high rate of hypoglycemia.

Though they do not endorse any particular discharge medication algorithm, ADA guidelines recommend measurement of hemoglobin A1C during the hospitalization, if not done in the last 3 months, to assist with discharge medication planning.[7]

Taking into account her moderately uncontrolled DM, you discharge her on her home oral antihyperglycemic agents as well as 50% of her hospital daily dose of insulin.

A 19-year-old female with type I DM presents to the ED with 3 days of symptoms consistent with viral gastroenteritis. Given poor oral intake, she stopped taking her insulin for fear of hypoglycemia. This morning she noted blood sugars of 400 mg/dL with positive urine ketones on home testing. In the ED, her blood sugar remains 400 mg/dL, and she has an arterial pH of 7.27 and an anion gap of 14 mEq/L. The ED calls you to admit her to the ICU for treatment of DKA. Upon your initial assessment, the patient is alert and hemodynamically stable; you diagnose her with uncomplicated moderate DKA and wonder if she needs to go to the ICU for an intravenous insulin infusion or if you can manage her with subcutaneous (SC) insulin on the general medical floor.

---

[7]See footnote 2.

In patients with uncomplicated DKA, is SC insulin a reasonable alternative to IV insulin?

In such patients, SC insulin has similar outcomes at possibly lower cost.

The use of SC lispro insulin and IV regular insulin were compared in a prospective randomized open-label trial of 40 patients with uncomplicated DKA (without persistent hypotension, loss of consciousness, acute myocardial infarction, heart failure, end-stage renal disease, anasarca, dementia, or pregnancy) at two urban US hospitals.[8]

The SC group (20 patients) was admitted to the general medical or step-down floor and treated with SC insulin lispro (0.3 unit/kg followed by 0.1 unit/kg/h) until resolution of hyperglycemia (blood glucose <250 mg/dL), followed by 0.05 to 0.1 unit/kg/h until resolution of ketoacidosis (bicarbonate ≥18 mEq/L and venous pH >7.3). Fingerstick glucose levels were checked hourly. The IV group (20 patients) was admitted to the ICU and treated with IV regular insulin (0.1 units/kg followed by 0.1 unit/kg/h) until resolution of hyperglycemia, followed by 0.05 to 0.1 unit/kg/h until resolution of ketoacidosis. Fingerstick glucose levels were checked every 2 hours.

Main outcomes were time to resolution of hyperglycemia and ketoacidosis, respectively, as well as frequency of hypoglycemia (blood glucose ≤60 mg/dL). Secondary outcomes included length of hospitalization and cost of treatment. There was no difference between SC and IV groups in terms of time to resolution of hyperglycemia (7 ± 3 vs. 7 ± 2 hours; $P = .29$) or ketoacidosis (10 ± 3 vs. 11 ± 4 hours; $P = .87$). Rates of hypoglycemia were equivalent (5% vs. 5%; P-value not recorded) and length of hospitalization was also similar (4 ± 1 vs. 4 ± 2 days; $P = .14$). Cost of treatment was lower for the SC group ($8801 ± 5549 vs. $14,429 ± 5243; $P < .01$).

Caveats include small sample size and number of study sites, more frequent glucose checks in the SC compared to the IV group, as well as confounding of cost data by different locations of care across groups. A meta-analysis including this study and four other small randomized trials of patients with mild to moderate DKA[9] found treatment with SC and IV insulin to have similar outcomes in terms of time to resolution of

---

[8]Umpierrez GE, et al. Efficacy of subcutaneous insulin lispro versus continuous intravenous regular insulin for the treatment of patients with diabetic ketoacidosis. *Am J Med.* 2004;117:291-296.

[9]Andrade-Castellanos CA, et al. Subcutaneous rapid-acting insulin analogues for diabetic ketoacidosis. *Cochrane Database Syst Rev.* 2016;(1):CD011281.

DKA and incidence of hypoglycemia. The ADA finds that in the absence of critical illness or obtundation, SC insulin may be a "safer and more cost-effective" option than IV insulin for mild to moderate DKA.[10]

Given her uncomplicated DKA, you opt to admit the patient to the floor for treatment with SC insulin. With this treatment, her labs normalize, her diet is advanced, and she is transitioned to long-acting insulin without any complications.

KEY LEARNING POINTS

1. A glucose range of 140 to 180 mg/dL is a recommended glycemic target for the majority of inpatients.
2. Sole use of SSI is discouraged, as it results in higher blood sugars than basal-bolus insulin.
3. Discharge medication algorithms based on hemoglobin A1C can lead to improved outpatient glycemic control.
4. Compared to IV insulin, SC insulin has similar outcomes at possibly lower cost in uncomplicated DKA.

---

[10]See footnote 2.

UPPER GASTROIN-TESTINAL BLEED

Kirsten Courtade, MD,
Jonathan Bortinger, MD

The ED calls you for an admission. The patient is a 51-year-old woman who began vomiting 2 days ago after several of her coworkers had the same symptoms. Prior to presentation, she vomited a small volume of "coffee ground" emesis. In the ED, her vitals are HR 75 bpm, BP 122/60 mm Hg, RR 16/min, and oxygen saturation 100% on room air. Labs are remarkable for Hgb 12.5 g/dL, BUN 10 mg/dL, and Cr 0.8 mg/dL. After an antiemetic, she is able to tolerate oral intake and wants to be discharged home. The ED physician asks you if she needs to be admitted for further treatment or monitoring.

Which patients with upper gastrointestinal bleed (UGIB) can be discharged without admission?

Patients with a Glasgow-Blatchford score (GBS) score of 0 can be safely managed in the outpatient setting.

The GBS is a risk stratification tool for UGIB based on gender, presentation (syncope, melena), hemodynamic (HR, SBP), lab (BUN, Hgb), and past medical history (hepatic disease, cardiac disease). It has been validated to predict the need for blood transfusion, endoscopic treatment, or surgery for UGIB.[1] A prospective study at four UK hospitals was designed to test the hypothesis that those with the lowest GBS (0) could be safely discharged from the ED without need for intervention (defined as blood transfusion, endoscopic treatment, or surgery) or

---

[1]Blatchford O, Murray WR, Blatchford M. A risk score to predict need for treatment for upper-gastrointestinal haemorrhage. *Lancet*. 2000;356(9238):1318-1321.

mortality.[2] In phase 1 of the study, 676 patients presenting with UGIB were evaluated (prospectively for 3-12 months at three hospitals, retrospectively for 3 months at one hospital). None of the 105 (16%) patients with a GBS of 0 required intervention or died after inpatient monitoring.

In phase 2, patients with GBS 0 were not hospitalized unless they had another indication for admission. Of 491 patients identified with UGIB, 123 had a GBS of 0, of whom, 84 were not hospitalized. Nonadmitted patients were followed with outpatient endoscopy or, in absence of endoscopy, by chart review or discussion with their family physician. Out of 123 patients with a GBS of 0, none required intervention. One of these patients died due to causes unrelated to their UGIB. Using GBS to identify the lowest risk patients could therefore avoid unnecessary admissions. Caveats include a somewhat small and homogenous population.

The 2012 American College of Gastroenterology (ACG) peptic ulcer guidelines note that discharge from the ED "may be considered" if GBS is 0.[3] Subsequent studies[4,5] suggest that patients with GBS ≤1 may also be good candidates for outpatient management due to low risk of mortality or need for intervention.

You advise the ED physician that the patient has a GBS score of 0 and is therefore at very low risk of adverse event or needing endoscopic therapy. You both agree that she can be discharged to follow-up with her primary care doctor.

A 70-year-old man with hypertension, prior stroke, and arthritis presents with melena and anemia. His vitals are stable. Labs are notable for Hgb 7.2 g/dL. You are suspicious that his bleed is from an upper source, but consider the possibility that this could in fact be a lower gastrointestinal bleed (LGIB). You wonder how you can determine that before the gastroenterology consultant arrives.

[2]Stanley AJ, et al. Outpatient management of patients with low-risk upper-gastrointestinal haemorrhage: multicentre validation and prospective evaluation. *Lancet.* 2009;373(9657):42-47.

[3]Laine L, Jensen DM. Management of patients with ulcer bleeding. *Am J Gastroenterol.* 2012;107(3):345-360.

[4]Laursen SB, et al. Performance of new thresholds of the Glasgow Blatchford Score in managing patients with upper gastrointestinal bleeding. *Clin Gastroenterol Hepatol.* 2015;13(1):115-121.

[5]Stanley AJ, et al. Comparison of risk scoring systems for patients presenting with upper gastrointestinal bleeding: international multicentre prospective study. *Br Med J.* 2017;356:i6432.

How accurate are signs, symptoms, and labs at distinguishing UGIB from LGIB?

Melena on examination and elevated blood urea nitrogen (BUN)/Cr ratio can be helpful in distinguishing an upper from lower source of bleeding. Nasogastric (NG) lavage with blood or coffee grounds, if present, makes UGIB much more likely, but false negatives are common.

A 2012 meta-analysis[6] assessed published studies regarding the diagnostic accuracy of signs and symptoms to differentiate UGIB and LGIB. Studies were selected if they involved patients with apparent GIB presenting to the ED or requiring hospitalization. Exclusion criteria included studies of primarily inpatients or children. Twenty-five studies met inclusion criteria. Sensitivity, specificity, +LRs (likelihood ratios), and −LRs were calculated.

Several features reliably rule in UGIB, including melena detected on clinical examination or observed by a clinician (+LR 25, 95% CI 4-174), NG lavage demonstrating blood or coffee ground material (+LR 9.6, 95% CI 4.0-23.0), and BUN/Cr ratio >30 (+LR 7.5, 95% CI 2.8-12.0). Other elements of history and physical are moderately helpful in determining if the patient has an UGIB, including prior history of UGIB (+LR 6.2, 95% CI 2.8-14.0) or patient report of melena (+LR ranging 5.1-5.9 in two studies). Of note, the absence of these features is not diagnostically useful to rule out UGIB.

Factors decreasing the likelihood of UGIB include clots in stool (+LR 0.05, 95% CI 0.01-0.38) and prior LGIB (+LR 0.17, 95% CI 0.09-0.35). NG lavage without blood or coffee ground material is only marginally helpful for ruling out UGIB (+LR 0.58, 95% CI 0.49-0.70). The resultant risk of falsely ruling out UGIB has led the ESGE to recommend against routine NG lavage in UGIB (strong recommendation, moderate quality evidence).[7]

You visualize melena during your examination and his BUN/Cr ratio is 35, both strongly suggesting UGIB rather than LGIB. He is resuscitated and scheduled for esophagogastroduodenoscopy (EGD). Prior to admission, the ED physician started a continuous infusion of proton pump inhibitor (PPI). You consider transitioning this to IV bolus dosing.

---

[6]Srygley FD, et al. Does this patient have a severe upper gastrointestinal bleed? *J Am Med Assoc.* 2012;307(10):1072-1079.

[7]Gralnek IM, et al. Diagnosis and management of nonvariceal upper gastrointestinal hemorrhage; European Society of Gastrointestinal Endoscopy (ESGE) Guideline. *Endoscopy.* 2015;47(10):a1-a46.

How do outcomes compare between intermittent dosing and continuous infusion of PPI in peptic ulcer disease?

Intermittent dosing of PPI is noninferior to continuous infusion.

Several studies have compared intermittent PPI dosing to continuous infusion. A 2014 meta-analysis included 13 randomized control trials of UGIB patients who were found to have high-risk ulcers (active bleeding, nonbleeding visible vessels, and ulcers with adherent clot) that were successfully managed endoscopically.[8] Intermittent dosing in included studies varied—notably, four trials used oral PPI. Continuous infusion was uniformly 80 mg IV bolus followed by 8 mg/h for 72 hours. The primary outcome was rebleeding at 7 days, and secondary outcomes included rebleeding at 3 and 30 days, mortality, transfusion, and hospital length of stay. This meta-analysis was designed as a noninferiority study with a predefined absolute risk difference of 3%.

Patients who received intermittent dosing had a lower risk of the primary outcome (RR 0.72, upper boundary of one-sided 95% CI 0.97; *P*-value not reported), and all secondary outcomes were also noninferior. Caveats include variable quality (e.g., lack of blinding) of a few trials.

> You transition the patient's PPI to intermittent IV dosing. The gastroenterology consultant performs an EGD that demonstrates a gastric ulcer with a visible vessel treated with endoscopic therapy including clips. The patient is asymptomatic and his repeat Hgb value is 7.4 g/dL. You wonder whether he should receive a red blood cell (RBC) transfusion.

What is an appropriate threshold for RBC transfusion in patients presenting with UGIB?

A restrictive (Hgb 7 g/dL) transfusion threshold is superior to a liberal (Hgb 9 g/dL) one.

Investigators performed a randomized controlled trial in 921 adults presenting to a single Spanish hospital with hematemesis, bloody NG

---

[8]Sachar H, Vaidya K, Laine L. Intermittent vs continuous proton pump inhibitor therapy for high-risk bleeding ulcers: a systematic review and meta-analysis. *JAMA Intern Med.* 2014;174(11):1755-1762.

aspirate, and/or melena confirmed by hospital staff.[9] Patients were excluded from the trial if they had massive exsanguinating hemorrhage, very low risk of complications (Rockall score of 0 with Hgb >12 g/dL), acute coronary syndrome, a recent history of trauma or surgery, LGIB, or transfusion within the previous 90 days.

Patients were randomized either to a restrictive (Hgb threshold 7 g/dL, target 7-9 g/dL) or liberal (Hgb threshold 9 g/dL, target 9-11 g/dL) transfusion strategy. RBC transfusion was permitted above the transfusion threshold if the patient required surgical intervention, experienced massive hemorrhage, or developed signs and symptoms of significant anemia; all other transfusions were deemed protocol violations. After randomization, all patients underwent EGD within the first 6 hours. The primary outcome was death from any cause within 45 days. Secondary outcomes included further bleeding (hematemesis or melena with hemodynamic instability or abrupt drop in Hgb).

Mortality was lower in the restrictive group (5% vs. 9%, HR 0.55, 95% CI 0.33-0.92; $P = .02$), as was risk of rebleeding (10% vs. 16%, HR 0.62, 95% CI 0.43-0.91; $P = .01$). The benefits of a restrictive strategy were particularly pronounced among cirrhotics. Those with Child-Pugh class A or B disease had lower mortality (HR 0.30, 95% CI 0.11-0.85; $P = .02$) and rebleeding (HR 0.53, 95% CI 0.27-0.94; $P = .04$). Nine percent of the restrictive group had protocol violation blood transfusions. Caveats include the rapid timeline for EGD (which may not be feasible in all settings), the high rate of protocol violations in the restrictive group, and the exclusion of those with massive exsanguination and acute coronary syndrome.

The 2015 ESGE guidelines for management of nonvariceal hemorrhage recommends a restrictive transfusion threshold to target Hgb between 7 to 9 g/dL unless significant comorbidities influence a clinician to target a higher threshold (strong recommendation, moderate quality of evidence).[10] The American Society for Gastrointestinal Endoscopy (ASGE) also cites this trial in recommending a target Hgb of 7 to 8 g/dL in treatment of variceal hemorrhage.[11] This trial provides additional support to the 2012 ACG clinical guideline that blood

---

[9]Villanueva C, et al. Transfusion strategies for acute upper gastrointestinal bleeding. *N Engl J Med.* 2013;368(1):11-21.

[10]See footnote 7.

[11]Hwang JH, et al. The role of endoscopy in the management of variceal hemorrhage. *Gastrointest Endosc.* 2014;80(2):221-227.

transfusions should target hemoglobin ≥7 g/dL in patients with ulcer bleeding (conditional recommendation, low- to moderate-quality evidence).[12]

> You adopt a restrictive strategy and decide not to administer RBC transfusion. You are currently holding the patient's home low-dose aspirin, which he takes for secondary prophylaxis after a remote stroke. He recognizes that aspirin can be harmful to his GI tract but is anxious about being off the medication for too long. He asks when he can safely resume it.

What are the risks and benefits of resuming low-dose aspirin for treatment or secondary prophylaxis of cardiovascular disease after achieving hemostasis of peptic ulcer bleeding?

Resuming low-dose aspirin in this setting is associated with a higher risk of rebleeding but lower all-cause mortality.

To answer this question, investigators performed a double-blind, randomized, controlled noninferiority trial of patients with UGIB (melena or hematemesis) at a single Chinese center.[13] Prior to presentation, all 156 patients had been taking aspirin (≤325 mg daily) for treatment or secondary prophylaxis of cardiovascular disease. All patients were treated with continuous infusion of PPI and achieved successful endoscopic hemostasis of high-risk peptic ulcer disease (active bleeding, visible vessel, or adherent clot). Immediately after endoscopy, patients were randomized to either resume aspirin (at a dose of 80 mg daily) or placebo for 8 weeks. Patients were excluded if they were receiving anticoagulants, steroids, or nonsteroidal anti-inflammatory drugs. The primary outcome was recurrent peptic ulcer bleeding within 30 days with a 10% noninferiority margin. Secondary outcomes included all-cause mortality and transfusion.

The rate of rebleeding within 30 days was nonequivalent between the aspirin and placebo groups (10.3% vs. 5.4%, risk difference 4.9%, 95% CI -3.6-13.4%; *P*-value not reported). Aspirin was associated with a lower rate of all-cause mortality at 30 days (1.3% vs. 9%, HR 0.2, 95%

---

[12]See footnote 3.

[13]Sung JJ, et al. Continuation of low-dose aspirin therapy in peptic ulcer bleeding: a randomized trial. *Ann Intern Med.* 2010;152(1):1-9.

CI 0.05-0.90; *P*-value not reported) and 8 weeks (1.3% vs. 12.9%, HR 0.2, 95% CI 0.06-0.60; *P*-value not reported). Caveats include the trial's small size and the lack of stratification by aspirin prophylaxis and/or treatment indication.

In their peptic ulcer disease guidelines, the ACG recommends restarting aspirin for secondary prophylaxis "as soon as possible after bleeding ceases in most patients: ideally within 1 to 3 days and certainly within 7 days" (conditional recommendation, moderate-quality evidence).[14]

> After discussing the increased risk of bleeding with lower mortality, you and the patient both feel comfortable resuming aspirin for secondary prophylaxis the following day.

KEY LEARNING POINTS

1. Patients with UGIB and GBS of 0 can be safely discharged with outpatient follow-up.
2. Melena (especially if visualized on examination) and an elevated BUN/Cr ratio can help distinguish UGIB from LGIB. Due to a high false-negative rate, routine NG lavage is no longer recommended for this purpose.
3. Intermittent PPI dosing is noninferior to continuous infusion in bleeding peptic ulcer disease.
4. In the absence of exsanguinating hemorrhage or acute coronary syndrome, a restrictive transfusion threshold (hgb 7 g/dL) is associated with lower mortality and rebleeding risk than a liberal (hgb 9 g/dL) transfusion threshold.
5. The resumption of low-dose aspirin for secondary cardiovascular prevention after an UGIB is associated with a higher risk of rebleeding but lower all-cause mortality.

---

[14]See footnote 3.

ACUTE LIVER INJURY AND FAILURE

Andrew Junkin, MD,
Joy J. Liu, MD

A 47-year-old woman with hypertension presents to the ED with 1 day of nausea, vomiting, anorexia, and right upper quadrant pain. She reports moderate to heavy drinking for many years, with a recent increase due to job-related stress. She is mildly tachycardic with epigastric tenderness and mild scleral icterus. Initial labs show WBC 16 k/μL, AST 110 units/L, ALT 35 units/L, alkaline phosphatase 80 units/L, TBili 4.4 mg/dL, PT 18.5 s, and INR 1.8. She is admitted for presumed alcoholic hepatitis and subsequently rules out for concomitant infection. Despite aggressive nutritional support, she continues to have severe disease based on her persistently elevated Maddrey discriminant function (MDF). You wonder if you should treat her with glucocorticoids.

Which patients with alcoholic hepatitis should be treated with glucocorticoids?

Patients with alcoholic hepatitis should be treated if the MDF score ≥32.

A 2015 network meta-analysis[1] assessed the role of glucocorticoids in patients with alcoholic hepatitis. This study included adults with severe alcoholic hepatitis (defined as MDF score ≥ 32 and/or hepatic encephalopathy) and was comprised of 22 randomized controlled trials (2621 patients) with a primary outcome of 4-week mortality. Glucocorticoids, pentoxifylline, and N-acetylcysteine (NAC) administered alone or in

---

[1]Singh S, et al. Comparative effectiveness of pharmacological interventions for severe alcoholic hepatitis: a systematic review and network meta-analysis. *Gastroenterology*. 2015;149(4):958-970.

combination for ≥4 weeks were compared to each other or placebo. Compared to placebo, short-term mortality was lower among patients receiving glucocorticoids alone (RR 0.54, 95% CI 0.39-0.73; no *P*-value reported) or in combination with pentoxifylline (RR 0.53, 95% CI 0.36-0.78; no *P*-value reported) or NAC (RR 0.15, 95% CI 0.05-0.39; no *P*-value reported). Study caveats include heterogeneity in studies (I^2 = 50% for corticosteroid versus placebo comparisons).

The American Association for the Study of Liver Diseases (AASLD) recommends that patients with MDF ≥32 receive a course of prednisolone (1A recommendation).[2]

Based on her elevated MDF and the absence of contraindications, you initiate therapy with prednisolone.

Another patient on your service, a 55-year-old woman with diabetes, hypertension, and obesity presented with 5 days of nausea and anorexia and 3 days of constant, progressive right upper quadrant abdominal pain without radiation. She is 1 month into isoniazid treatment for latent tuberculosis. Her initial labs are notable for AST 126 units/L, ALT 183 units/L, alkaline phosphatase 180 units/L, TBili 2.5 mg/dL, PT 16.9 seconds, and INR 1.6.

A broad initial workup for her acute liver injury (ALI) rules out a number of causes including infiltrative, autoimmune, inflammatory, vascular, and many viral diseases (hepatitis A, hepatitis B, hepatitis C, cytomegalovirus, and Epstein-Barr virus). You strongly suspect isoniazid-related drug-induced liver injury (DILI), a diagnosis of exclusion, but wonder whether you should test for hepatitis E virus despite a lack of obvious risk factors.

Is it reasonable to test for hepatitis E virus in ALI?

If initial testing for etiology of ALI is unrevealing, it is reasonable to test for hepatitis E infection even in the absence of obvious risk factors.

Testing for hepatitis E in cases of ALI is rarely positive but may result in changes in diagnosis and management. A prospective study[3]

---

[2]O'Shea RS, et al. Alcoholic liver disease. *Hepatology.* 2010;51(1):307-328.
[3]Davern TJ, et al. Acute hepatitis e infection accounts for some cases of suspected drug-induced liver injury. *Gastroenterology.* 2011;141(5):1665-1672.e1-9.

of 318 suspected DILI patients evaluated hepatitis E serologies (IgM, IgG) in samples obtained at time of enrollment. Certain patients had reflexive polymerase chain reaction (PCR) testing. Nine (3%) tested positive for hepatitis E IgM, indicating acute hepatitis E infection, and four had hepatitis E viremia at the time of serum sample testing. Patients with hepatitis E IgM positivity were older ($P < .001$) and male ($P < .003$), and 2/9 patients had HIV. None had traditional risk factors, such as recent travel to endemic areas, recent contact with farm animals, or consumption of undercooked pork. A positive hepatitis E IgM changed the most likely diagnosis to hepatitis E in 7/9 cases on a repeat causality analysis by three independent reviewers. In 3/7 cases, a "definite" (>95% likelihood) diagnosis of acute hepatitis E infection–induced liver injury was made. This study is limited by the low number of positive cases but demonstrates that patients being evaluated for DILI could have acute hepatitis E as the true cause of ALI.

A retrospective case series[4] that examined patient characteristics in cases of hepatitis E identified at the Centers for Disease Control and Prevention (CDC) further supports testing patients who lack traditional risk factors. Between 2005 and 2012, 26 positive cases of either acute or chronic hepatitis E infection were identified. Sixty-nine percent were jaundiced, 58% reported not having traveled outside the United States in <2 months, and 27% were solid organ transplant recipients. Acute liver failure (ALF) developed in 3/26 patients. This study suggests nontravelers are at risk of hepatitis E infection, but was limited to samples sent to the CDC, so may not reflect the true prevalence of hepatitis E in the US population.

> Hepatitis E is tested for and ruled out, leaving DILI as the most likely diagnosis. The next morning, liver enzymes have risen to AST 210 units/L, ALT 1457 units/L, alkaline phosphatase 650 units/L, TBili 5.1 mg/dL, and INR 2.1. Examination reveals no evidence of hepatic encephalopathy, but she is now jaundiced. The patient and her family ask about the prognosis for her condition and how it might affect her treatment options.

---

[4]Drobeniuc J, et al. Laboratory-based surveillance for hepatitis E virus infection, United States, 2005–2012. *Emerg Infect Dis*. 2013;19(2):218-222.

What features of ALI portend a poor outcome (i.e., ALF, liver transplant, or death)?

Risk factors for poor outcomes in ALI include jaundice >3 days, INR ≥1.7, TBili ≥3.0 mg/dL, etiology other than acetaminophen, and serum acetaminophen level >60 mg/L (in patients with acetaminophen-induced ALI).

Risk Factors for Poor Outcome in ALI

Acetaminophen-Induced ALI	Non-acetaminophen-Induced ALI
1. Jaundice >3 days 2. Acetaminophen level >60 mg/L 3. TBili ≥3.0 mg/dL 4. Initial INR ≥1.7	1. Etiology (non-acetaminophen) 2. Jaundice >3 days 3. TBili ≥3.0 mg/dL 4. Initial INR ≥1.7

The Acute Liver Failure Study Group[5] prospectively studied 386 patients with severe ALI to evaluate predictors of a primary composite outcome of ALF, liver transplant, or death within 21 days of enrollment. Severe ALI was defined as meeting the consensus definition of ALI (INR ≥1.5, ALT ≥10× ULN, the absence of hepatic encephalopathy, and, if the etiology is non-acetaminophen-related, TBili ≥3.0 mg/dL, in a patient without a history of chronic liver disease) plus an INR ≥2.0 within 48 hours of enrollment.

Twenty-three percent progressed to the primary outcome. This outcome occurred more frequently in patients with non-acetaminophen-associated ALI than those with acetaminophen-associated ALI (40% vs. 7%; $P < .001$). Other risk factors for the primary outcome include jaundice >3 days ($P < .001$), TBili ≥3.0 mg/dL ($P < .001$), or INR ≥1.7 ($P < .001$) (see table above). Using these risk factors, the authors created a random forest model for prediction of progression to ALF, liver transplant, or death. When applied to a validation dataset of 163 patients with severe ALI, the model was moderately predictive (PPV 88% [28/32], NPV 67% [95/141]).

This study demonstrates that certain objective features in ALI are associated with progression to ALF, liver transplant, or death, and that patients with a non-acetaminophen ALI have a much more guarded prognosis.

---

[5]Koch DG, et al. The natural history of severe acute liver injury. *Am J Gastro.* 2017;112(9): 1389-1396.

Given the worrisome laboratory findings, you initiate discussion with a liver transplant center regarding transfer. The physician at the transplant center accepts the patient but warns that transfer may take 24 to 48 hours. The next day, the patient develops mild asterixis and takes longer to respond to questions. Given her development of grade I hepatic encephalopathy, she now meets criteria for ALF. The transplant center hepatology team suggests supportive pharmacologic treatment while urgent transfer is arranged during the next few hours.

Should patients with non-acetaminophen-induced ALF and early-stage coma grade receive N-acetylcysteine (NAC)?

In patients with drug-induced liver failure and early-stage coma grade, it is reasonable to administer NAC to improve transplant-free survival.

This question was examined by a 2009 randomized, double-blind trial that randomized 173 patients with non-acetaminophen-induced ALF to either NAC or placebo.[6] Patients were eligible if they met criteria for ALF (any degree of encephalopathy, INR ≥1.5, and illness <24 weeks duration) and were excluded for age >70 years, known or suspected acetaminophen overdose, hepatic ischemia ("shock liver"), septic shock, or imminent transplantation (<8 hours). Patients were stratified by severity of hepatic encephalopathy—mild (grades I-II) or severe (grades III-IV). The primary outcome was survival at 3 weeks, and secondary outcomes included rate of liver transplantation and transplant-free survival. Patient outcomes were censored at 1 year.

Survival at 3 weeks did not differ between the NAC and placebo groups (70% vs. 66%, respectively; $P = .283$). Rate of liver transplantation was not different across groups (35% for NAC vs. 45% for placebo; $P = .093$), but patients receiving NAC had significantly better transplant-free survival (40% vs. 27%; $P = .043$), a difference that persisted at 1 year. NAC led to improvements in transplant-free survival in patients presenting with mild ($P = .01$) but not severe ($P = .912$) hepatic encephalopathy. Approximately 58% of patients in the NAC group received the full 72-hour infusion, with the most common reasons for early discontinuation being death, decision to withdraw treatment, or liver transplantation.

---

[6]Lee WM, et al. Intravenous N-acetylcysteine improves transplant-free survival in early stage non-acetaminophen acute liver failure. *Gastroenterology.* 2009;137(3):856-864.

The AASLD advises that NAC may be beneficial for non-acetaminophen-induced ALF, and strongly recommends its use in DILI-induced ALF (grade I recommendation).[7]

You start NAC prior to transfer to the transplant center. A week later you receive follow-up from the accepting hepatologist that the patient is about to receive a deceased donor transplant that evening.

KEY LEARNING POINTS

1. Patients with alcoholic hepatitis should be treated with steroids if the MDF score ≥32.
2. If initial testing for etiology of ALI is unrevealing, it is reasonable to test for hepatitis E infection even in the absence of obvious risk factors.
3. Risk factors for poor outcomes in ALI include jaundice >3 days, INR ≥1.7, TBili ≥3.0 mg/dL, etiology other than acetaminophen, and serum acetaminophen level >60 mg/L (in patients with acetaminophen-induced ALI).
4. In patients with drug-induced liver failure and early-stage coma grade, it is reasonable to administer NAC to improve transplant-free survival.

[7]Lee WM, et al. *AASLD Position Paper: The Management of Acute Liver Failure*. Update 2011. AASLD. Available at: https://www.aasld.org/sites/default/files/guideline_documents/alfenhanced.pdf. Accessed April 5, 2018.

ACUTE CORONARY SYNDROME

13

Zahir Kanjee, MD, MPH,
Joshua M. Liao, MD, MSc

The ED pages you regarding two chest pain admissions for possible acute coronary syndrome (ACS). The ED physician confirms that evaluations with ECG and troponin have been initiated on both patients, and neither has an ST-elevation myocardial infarction (STEMI). You assess the patients to see whether they have non-ST elevation (NSTE)-ACS such as unstable angina or NSTEMI.

Is there an evidence-based approach to differentiating NSTE-ACS from noncardiac causes of chest pain on initial evaluation?

Clinical prediction tools can outperform individual historical, examination, and ECG findings. These tools (e.g., HEART and TIMI scores) can be helpful in differentiating NSTE-ACS from noncardiac chest pain.

This question was studied in a 2015 systematic review[1] that evaluated all potentially relevant articles from January 1995 to July 2015. Authors included studies meeting three criteria: (1) presentation to the ED with suspected ACS, (2) clear descriptions of diagnostic testing (including history, physical, ECG, overall assessment, and clinical prediction tools including the HEART score and the TIMI score (Table 13.1), and (3) adequate listing of outcomes (either hospital discharge diagnosis or subsequent significant cardiovascular event).

To focus primarily on using available tools to differentiate patients at point of first contact, the review excluded studies (1) in which

---

[1]Faranoff AC, et al. Does this patient with chest pain have acute coronary syndrome? The rational clinical examination systematic review. *J Am Med Assoc.* 2015;314(18):1955-1965.

TABLE 13.1

Clinical Decision Tools to Assess ACS

Clinical Prediction Tool	Variable	High-Risk Score Value	+LR for ACS	Low-Risk Score Value	+LR for ACS
HEART score Scores five variables on scale of 0-2 to give score 0-10	History: 0 points for history incompatible with ACS, 1 point for history potentially compatible with ACS, and 2 points for history strongly suggestive of ACS EKG: 0 points for normal ECG, 1 point for ECG with nonspecific repolarization abnormalities, and 2 points for ECG with ST depression or transient ST elevation Age: 0 points for < 45 years, 1 point for 45-65 years, and 2 points for > 65 years Risk factors: 0 points for no risk factors, 1 point for 1-2 risk factors, and 2 points for ≥ 3 risk factors or known CAD Troponin: 0 points for normal troponin level, 1 point for 1-3 × upper limit of normal, and 2 points for >3 × upper limit of normal	7-10	13 (95% CI 7.0-24)	0-3	0.20 (95% CI 0.13-0.30)
TIMI score Assesses for presence of seven variables to give score 0-7	Age ≥ 65 years ≥ 3 cardiac risk factors Known CAD Aspirin use ≥ 2 episodes of angina in preceding 24 hours ST-segment elevation or depression ≥ 0.5 mm Elevation in cardiac biomarkers	5-7	6.8 (95% CI 5.2-8.9)	0-1	0.31 (95% CI 0.23-0.43)

ACS, acute coronary syndrome; CAD, coronary artery disease; LR, likelihood ratio.

Data from Backus BE, Six AJ, Kelder JC, et al. A prospective validation of the HEART score for chest pain patients at the emergency department. *Int J Cardiol.* 2013;168(3):2154; Antman EM, et al. The TIMI Risk Score for unstable angina/non-ST elevation MI: A method for prognostication and therapeutic decision making. *J Am Med Assoc.* 2000;284(7)835-842; and Faranoff AC, et al. Does this patient with chest pain have acute coronary syndrome? The rational clinical examination systematic review. *J Am Med Assoc.* 2015;314(18);1955-1965.

assessment was initiated after acquisition of serial ECGs/troponins, (2) among patients at disproportionately high, intermediate, or low probability of ACS, and (3) using high-sensitivity troponin assays, which were not routinely available in the United States at the time of study. Fifty-eight articles were included in the final analysis.

The authors found several commonly used predictors of ACS to be of mild to moderate utility. Mildly helpful to rule in ACS were a history of an abnormal stress test (+LR 3.1, 95% CI 2.0-4.7) and pain radiating to both arms (+LR 2.6, 95% CI 1.8-3.7). More useful were ST depression (+LR 5.3, 95% CI 2.1-8.6) or "ischemic" ECG (+LR 3.6, 95% CI 1.6-5.7). However, each of these findings was limited by poor sensitivity and resultant poor ability to rule out ACS. Clinicians' overall impression of whether a patient had ACS prior to seeing their ECG and troponin was somewhat more diagnostic ("definite" ACS + LR 4.0, 95% CI 2.5-6.6; "definitely not" ACS + LR 0.36, 95% CI 0.05-2.8).

Formal decision tools were superior for predicting ACS. A high HEART score (7-10) was associated with +LR 13 (95% CI 7.0-24) for ACS, high TIMI score (5-7) with +LR 6.8 (95% CI 5.2-9.0). Low HEART score (0-3) was associated with +LR 0.20 (95% CI 0.13-0.30), low TIMI score (0-1) with +LR 0.31 (95% CI 0.23-0.43). Study caveats include the use of revascularization, which can be affected by measurement bias, as an outcome in many studies.

The first patient is a 44-year-old man with hypertension who presents with a single episode of chest pain. The episode was potentially consistent with ACS by history. His only medication is amlodipine and aspirin. His ECG has nonspecific repolarization abnormalities, and his troponin is negative. You find him to have a TIMI score of 1 and a HEART score of 3 (both low risk). Based on his low risk for ACS, you discharge him from observation after a second troponin and ECG several hours later. Working with his primary care physician, you arrange for an outpatient stress test within 48 hours of discharge.

The second patient is a 67-year-old man with a hyperlipidemia, hypertension, and family history of early coronary disease who presents with three episodes that are strongly suggestive of ACS by history in the last 24 hours. After two sublingual nitroglycerin tablets, his pain is resolved. His medication list includes hydrochlorothiazide, pravastatin, and aspirin. ECG shows 1 mm ST depressions in anterior leads as well as nonspecific T-wave inversions. His repeat troponin

(continued)

is within normal limits. You calculate his TIMI and HEART scores as 5 and 8, respectively (both high risk). You diagnose this patient with unstable angina and admit him to an inpatient telemetry bed.

You start to think about approaches to revascularization. You note the patient does not have any immediate indication for catheterization, such as refractory angina or hemodynamic or electrical instability. You therefore consider a routine invasive strategy (up-front angiography with intent to intervene) or an ischemia-guided strategy (medical management for all but the highest prognostic risk, with routine stress test and reservation of catheterization for those who fail therapy or have a positive stress).

Which patients with NSTE-ACS should receive which revascularization strategy?

Both routine invasive or ischemia-guided approaches are potentially reasonable for patients with NSTE-ACS, though the invasive strategy is recommended for high-risk patients.

A meta-analysis has compared routine invasive versus ischemia-guided strategies in NSTE-ACS patients.[2] The authors included all three randomized studies with available long-term outcomes, comprising 5467 patients. The primary outcome was cardiovascular death or nonfatal MI. At 5 years, this outcome occurred less frequently in the invasive group than the ischemia-guided group (14.7% vs. 17.9%, HR 0.81; CI 0.71-0.93; P = .002). The benefits from the invasive strategy were particularly notable among those deemed to be at highest risk (i.e., those with a greater number of the following attributes: older age, diabetes, hypertension, ST-segment depression, and elevated body mass index). Since troponin values were not available in all patients in all studies due to evolving use of biomarkers at the time, this was not included in the risk scoring. This meta-analysis has two main limitations regarding heterogeneity of interventions across the studies: first, studies had variable timing for catheterization in the invasive arms (ranging from 24-48 h in 1 to 7 days in another) and second, one study's ischemia-guided approach did not necessitate a predischarge stress test.

---

[2]Fox KA, et al. Long-term outcome of a routine versus selective invasive strategy in patients with non-ST-segment elevation acute coronary syndrome: a meta-analysis of individual patient data. *J Am Coll Cardiol*. 2010;55(22):2435-2445.

The 2014 American Heart Association (AHA)/American College of Cardiology (ACC) NSTE-ACS guidelines[3] recommend an early invasive strategy for those at high clinical risk (including changes in troponin or new ST depression on ECG, among others; recommendation class I, level of evidence B).

Based on his high risk for adverse outcomes, an early invasive strategy is selected. At catheterization, the patient is found to have a 99% stenosis of his left anterior descending coronary artery and receives a drug eluting stent (DES). On the day of discharge, you discuss medication changes from his preadmission list, noting that you changed his home statin, pravastatin 20 mg daily, to atorvastatin 80 mg daily. He asks why you made this change.

Is there a benefit to high-dose versus low-dose statin in the setting of ACS?

Intensive lipid-lowering therapy with high-dose statins is associated with better outcomes than less intense therapy in the ACS setting.

Two clinical trials addressing this question are worth noting. The first is the MIRACL study,[4] a double-blind, placebo-controlled, international randomized trial of 3068 adults with unstable angina or non-Q wave MI. Patients with very high (>270-310 mg/dL) total cholesterol or those using other lipid-lowering agents (besides niacin) were excluded. Patients were randomized to receive either atorvastatin 80 mg or placebo daily within 24 to 96 hours of hospital admission for 16 weeks. The primary outcome (death, nonfatal MI, cardiac arrest with resuscitation, and emergency rehospitalization for recurrent ischemia) occurred in 14.8% in the atorvastatin group compared with 17.4% in the placebo group (P = .048). MIRACL showed that statin therapy could be beneficial acutely in ACS and that it should be begun prior to discharge.

---

[3]Amsterdam EA, et al. 2014 AHA/ACC guideline for the management of patients with non-ST-elevation acute coronary syndromes: executive summary. *Circulation.* 2014;130(25):2354-2394.
[4]Schwartz GG, et al. Effects of atorvastatin on early recurrent ischemic events in acute coronary syndromes: the MIRACL study: a randomized controlled trial. *J Am Med Assoc.* 2001;285(13):1711-1718.

This notion was further advanced through the PROVE IT-TIMI 22 study.[5] This double-blind, double-dummy, international clinical trial randomized 4162 adults hospitalized for ACS within the prior 10 days to either atorvastatin 80 mg or pravastatin 40 mg orally daily, with pravastatin increased to 80 mg daily in a blinded manner if low density lipoprotein (LDL) remained >125 mg/dL. Patients with very elevated total cholesterol (>240 mg/dL, or >200 if taking lipid-lowering therapy) and those already on statin therapy at 80 mg/day at the time of the index event were excluded.

At 2 years, the primary outcome (death from any cause, MI, unstable angina requiring rehospitalization, revascularization >30 days from randomization, and stroke) occurred in a lower proportion of the atorvastatin group (22.4% vs. 26.3%; $P = .005$). The benefit was seen as early as 30 days from randomization. PROVE IT showed that a high-dose statin, as opposed to a moderate dose, had early and persistent effects in the post-ACS setting. The 2014 AHA/ACC NSTE-ACS guidelines[6] recommend high-intensity statins for all NSTE-ACS patients in the absence of contraindications (recommendation class I, level of evidence A).

After explaining the benefits of high-intensity therapy to him, you discharge him on atorvastatin 80 mg orally daily in place of his home statin. His cardiologist advises him to continue taking aspirin and ticagrelor for long-term dual antiplatelet therapy (DAPT). Thirteen months later, he re-presents with acute upper gastrointestinal bleeding requiring transfusion and admission. He has remained on ticagrelor and aspirin and has had no further cardiovascular events or angina. This is his first episode of bleeding, and you suspect that his prolonged DAPT may have contributed to his risk. The endoscopist asks you whether there are any data to guide risk-benefit decisions about prolonged DAPT.

What are the risks and benefits of prolonged DAPT?

Prolonged DAPT is associated with less stent thrombosis and cardiovascular and cerebrovascular events. It is also associated with a higher bleeding risk than monotherapy.

---

[5]Cannon CP, et al. Intensive versus moderate lipid lowering with statins after acute coronary syndromes. *N Engl J Med.* 2004;350(15):1495-1504.
[6]See footnote 3.

Investigators have attempted to assess the effect of prolonged (i.e., > 12 months) DAPT therapy. The most prominent trial is the DAPT study, [7] an international randomized controlled trial which evaluated patients ≥ 18 years who had received a DES and demonstrated good adherence to 12 months of aspirin plus either clopidogrel or prasugrel as DAPT without adverse cardiovascular or cerebrovascular events or bleeding. Patients on therapeutic anticoagulation were excluded. After 12 months of DAPT, 9961 patients continued aspirin but were randomized to either continue their second antiplatelet agent or to take a placebo for 18 additional months. Coprimary outcomes were definite/probable stent thrombosis or major cardiovascular/cerebrovascular events (a composite of death, MI, or stroke). The primary safety outcome was moderate or severe bleeding.

The prolonged DAPT group had less stent thrombosis (0.4% vs. 1.4%, HR 0.29, CI 0.17-0.48; $P < .001$) and fewer major adverse cardiovascular/cerebrovascular events (4.3% vs. 5.9%, HR 0.71, 95% CI 0.59-0.85; $P < .001$). The rate of moderate or severe bleeding was higher in the continued DAPT group (2.5% vs. 1.5%, HR 1.61, 95% CI 1.21-2.16; $P = .001$). Of note, all-cause mortality was higher in the continued DAPT group (2.0% vs. 1.5%; $P = .05$). *Post hoc*, the authors identified an imbalance in the prerandomization distribution of patients with cancer and found that excluding these patients led to mortality differences becoming nonsignificant and less pronounced. Caveats include a long run-in period that eliminated those with preceding adverse events from DAPT, limiting generalizability. These findings led to an update of AHA/ACC guidelines[8] which now suggest prolonged DAPT as an acceptable option (recommendation class IIb, level of evidence A). In a secondary analysis of DAPT trial data, researchers created and validated a risk calculator[9] to assist with comparing the risks and benefits of continuation of DAPT in those who have already tolerated 12 months of therapy. The score incorporates features such as age, diabetes, type and size of stent, and presence of heart failure, among others, to predict whether an individual patient is more likely to derive benefit (in terms of preventing ischemia) or harm (due to excessive bleeding) from prolonged DAPT.

---

[7]Mauri L, et al. Twelve or 30 months of dual antiplatelet therapy after drug-eluting stents. *N Engl J Med*. 2014;371(23):2155-2166.

[8]Levine GN, et al. 2016 ACC/AHA guideline focused update on duration of dual antiplatelet therapy in patients with coronary artery disease. *J Am Coll Cardiol*. 2016;68(10):1082-1115.

[9]Yeh RW, et al. Development and validation of a prediction rule for benefit and harm of dual antiplatelet therapy beyond one year after percutaneous coronary intervention: an analysis from the randomized dual antiplatelet therapy study. *J Am Med Assoc*. 2016;315(16):1735-1749.

You discuss the risks and benefits of DAPT with the patient and his cardiologist. Given his DAPT risk calculator score of -1 (associated with an unfavorable benefit/risk ratio for prolonged DAPT) and his gastrointestinal bleed, the patient and medical team all agree to discontinue the second antiplatelet agent.

KEY LEARNING POINTS

1. Clinical prediction tools can outperform individual historical, examination, and ECG findings. These tools (e.g., HEART and TIMI scores) can be helpful in differentiating NSTE-ACS from noncardiac chest pain.
2. Both routine invasive or ischemia-guided approaches are potentially reasonable for patients with NSTE-ACS, though the invasive strategy is recommended for high-risk patients.
3. Intensive lipid-lowering therapy with high-dose statins is associated with better outcomes than less intense therapy in the ACS setting.
4. Prolonged DAPT is associated with less stent thrombosis and cardiovascular and cerebrovascular events. It is also associated with a higher bleeding risk than monotherapy.

PNEUMONIA

Lauren Noll, MD,
Neha Deshpande, MD

The ED calls you regarding a 65-year-old man with a history of hypertension presenting with fever and cough. He is tachycardic to 125/min, with a respiratory rate of 35/min. Physical examination is notable for dullness to percussion and crackles over the right upper lung field, and his labs reveal a white blood cell count of 13,000/μL but are otherwise within normal limits. His chest radiograph demonstrates the following:

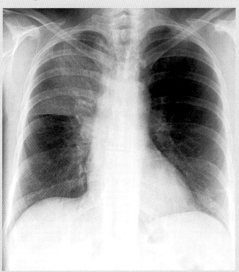

His clinical and imaging findings are consistent with pneumonia. He has not had any recent contact with the healthcare system. You discuss with the ED provider whether admission to the hospital is warranted.

Which patients diagnosed with community-acquired pneumonia (CAP) are suitable for outpatient treatment rather than hospital admission?

Patients who may be suitable for outpatient treatment can be identified using severity of illness scores and prognostic models, such as the Pneumonia Severity Index (PSI) and CURB-65.

This question was addressed in a 1997 study evaluating how treatment decisions could be standardized with a prognostic model of illness severity.[1] Using a derivation cohort of 14,199 inpatients with CAP, the authors identified 20 factors independently associated with mortality, each assigned point values based on the magnitude of association. This model, known as the PSI, produced five risk classes and was then tested on two validation cohorts consisting mostly of inpatients with a small cohort of outpatients (Table 14.1). Mortality did not differ within risk classes. For example, mortality ranged from 0.1% to 0.4% (class I), 0.6% to 0.7% (class II), and 0.9% to 2.8% (class III) (*P* > .05 for all).

Given barriers to the use of PSI (e.g., numerous variables and need for time-intensive calculation), a 2003 cohort study sought to derive a simpler model.[2] Based on British Thoracic Society (BTS) guidelines previously validated to identify patients with severe CAP, a derivation cohort of 1068 patients hospitalized with CAP was used to identify five variables independently associated with mortality. From these data, authors derived the CURB-65 model, which stratified patients into three classes according to mortality risk (Table 14.1). CURB-65 was then applied to an inpatient validation cohort and demonstrated no observed differences in mortality within risk classes between the derivation and validation cohorts. Despite the benefit of its simplicity for clinical use, the CURB-65 was derived and validated among inpatients only, potentially limiting its applicability in the outpatient setting.

While not substitutes for clinical judgment, Infectious Diseases Society of America (IDSA) guidelines support the use of these prognostic models for guiding risk stratification and identifying patients at the

---

[1]Fine MJ, et al. A prediction rule to identify low-risk patients with community-acquired pneumonia. *N Engl J Med.* 1997;336(4):243-250.
[2]Lim WS, et al. Defining community acquired pneumonia severity on presentation to hospital: an international derivation and validation study. *Thorax.* 2003;58(5):377-382.

TABLE 14.1

PSI and CURB-65 Prognostic Models

Prognostic Model	Variables		Risk Category	Suggested Treatment Site
Pneumonia Severity Index (PSI)	**Demographics:** Age:	**Points:**	Class I (<50)	Outpatient
	Men	Age (years)	Class II (50-70)	Outpatient
	Women	Age (years) -10		
	Nursing home resident	+10	Class III (71-90)	Outpatient vs. brief inpatient
	Comorbidities:			
	Neoplastic disease	+30		
	Liver disease	+20	Class IV (91-130)	Inpatient
	Congestive heart failure	+10		
	Cerebrovascular disease	+10		
	Renal disease	+10	Class V(>130)	Inpatient
	Physical examination/vitals:			
	Altered mental status	+20		
	Respiratory rate ≥30/min	+20		
	Systolic blood pressure <90 mm Hg	+20		
	Temperature <35°C or ≥40°C	+15		
	Pulse ≥125/min	+10		

(Continued)

TABLE 14.1

PSI and CURB-65 Prognostic Models

Prognostic Model	Variables		Risk Category	Suggested Treatment Site
	Labs/imaging:			
	Arterial pH <7.35	+30		
	BUN ≥30 mg/dL	+20		
	Sodium <130 mmol/L	+20		
	Glucose ≥250 mg/dL	+10		
	Hct <30%	+10		
	PaO$_2$ <60 mm Hg	+10		
	Pleural effusion	+10		
CURB-65	One point given for each: Confusion		Score 0-1: Mortality low (1.5%)	Outpatient
	Urea >19 mg/dL (>7 mmol/L) Respiratory rate ≥30/min Systolic blood pressure <90 mm Hg or Diastolic blood pressure ≤60 mm Hg		Score 2: Mortality intermediate (9.2%)	Outpatient vs. brief inpatient
	Age ≥65 years		Score 3 or more: Mortality high (22%)	Inpatient

PSI reprinted from Fine MJ, et al. A prediction rule to identify low-risk patients with community-acquired pneumonia. *N Engl J Med.* 1997;336(4):243-250, with permission. CURB-65 data from Lim WS, et al. Defining community acquired pneumonia severity on presentation to hospital: an international derivation and validation study. *Thorax.* 2003;58(5):377-382.

lowest risk of mortality who may be appropriate for outpatient treatment (strong recommendation; level I evidence).[3]

> The patient has no other comorbidities, laboratory, or imaging abnormalities, corresponding to an intermediate mortality risk based on PSI (class IV) and CURB-65 (2). The decision is made to admit the patient to the hospital for intravenous antibiotics. One hour later, he becomes hypotensive to 90/60 mmHg. After a 2L bolus of crystalloid, his systolic pressure improves to 110 mmHg, but he remains tachypneic and tachycardic. You discuss with the ED provider whether this patient needs ICU level of care.

What are strategies for identifying patients with CAP who would benefit from intensive care?

In addition to patients requiring vasopressors and/or mechanical ventilation, direct ICU admission is recommended for patients with ≥3 IDSA/American Thoracic Society (ATS) minor criteria for severe CAP.

A 2004 study evaluated nine prediction rules for ICU admission and mortality among patients with CAP.[4] The study prospectively enrolled 696 inpatients with CAP, 116 of whom (16.7%) were initially admitted to the ICU. The modified ATS rule demonstrated the highest sensitivity (69%, 95% CI 51%-77%) and specificity (97%, 95% CI 96%-99%) for predicting admission to the ICU. This rule was defined as two of three minor criteria on admission (systolic blood pressure[SBP] <90 mm Hg, multilobar involvement, PaO_2/FiO_2 ≤250) or one of two major criteria (need for mechanical ventilation, septic shock). The modified ATS rule was also shown to be most predictive of mortality, with a sensitivity of 94% (95% CI 83%-99%) and specificity of 93% (95% CI 91%-95%). Based on these results, the ATS rule was combined with previously validated CURB-65 criteria to form the IDSA/ATS major and minor criteria (Table 14.2).

A subsequent 2011 prospective observational study of 1062 patients with CAP evaluated whether these IDSA/ATS minor criteria predicted ICU admission, need for mechanical ventilation or vasopressor support,

---

[3]Mandell LA, et al. Infectious Diseases Society of America/American Thoracic Society consensus guidelines on the management of community-acquired pneumonia in adults. *Clin Infect Dis.* 2007;44(suppl 2):S27-S72.

[4]Ewig S, et al. Validation of predictive rules and indices of severity for community acquired pneumonia. *Thorax.* 2004;59(5):421-427.

TABLE 14.2

IDSA/ATS Criteria for Severe CAP

Major criteria:
Invasive mechanical ventilation
Vasopressor support
Minor criteria:
Respiratory rate ≥30 breaths/min
PaO_2/FiO_2 ratio ≤250
Multilobar infiltrates
Confusion
Uremia (BUN ≥20 mg/dL)
Leukopenia (WBC <4000 cells/mm³)
Thrombocytopenia (platelets <100,000 cells/mm³)
Hypothermia (<36°C)
Hypotension requiring fluid resuscitation

IDSA, Infectious Diseases Society of America; ATS, American Thoracic Society; CAP, community-acquired pneumonia.

Reprinted from Mandell LA, et al. Infectious Diseases Society of America/American Thoracic Society consensus guidelines on the management of community-acquired pneumonia in adults. *Clin Infect Dis.* 2007;44(suppl 2):S27-S72, with permission from Oxford University Press.

and 30-day mortality.[5] Each of the nine minor criteria (Table 14.2) were individually associated with these outcomes, and as a collective set, the IDSA/ATS minor criteria possessed area under the receiver operator characteristic curves of 0.85 (95% CI 0.82-0.88), 0.85 (95% CI 0.82-0.88), and 0.78 (95% CI 0.74-0.82) for need for mechanical ventilation or vasopressor support, ICU admission, and 30-day mortality, respectively.

These studies demonstrate the utility of the IDSA/ATS minor criteria for informing decisions about level of care by identifying patients at high risk of decompensation and death despite not immediately requiring mechanical ventilation or vasopressor support. IDSA guidelines suggest benefit to early ICU admission in patients with ≥3 minor criteria (moderate recommendation; level II evidence).[3]

---

[5]Chalmers JD, et al. Validation of the Infectious Diseases Society of America/American Thoracic Society minor criteria for intensive care unit admission in community acquired pneumonia patients without major criteria or contraindications to intensive care unit care. *Clin Infect Dis.* 2011;53(6):503-511.

The patient meets only two minor criteria for severe CAP, so he is admitted to the acute care floor. Based on IDSA guidelines, you start him on empiric treatment with IV ceftriaxone and azithromycin but also consider whether further workup is warranted to inform antibiotic choice.

Is there benefit to pathogen-directed versus empiric therapy for patients with CAP?

There is no mortality difference between pathogen-directed therapy and empiric therapy in patients with CAP.

A 1999 retrospective cohort study investigated the role of microbiological studies in the evaluation and treatment of patients with CAP.[6] Using a population of 184 hospitalized patients designated as having severe CAP (SCAP) or nonsevere CAP (NSCAP) based on ATS guidelines, authors examined response to antibiotic therapy. Nonresponders were defined as those with persistent fever, leukocytosis, or clinical deterioration within 24 hours to 5 days of hospitalization.

14% of patients did not respond to initial antibiotic regimens (6 with NSCAP vs. 19 with SCAP), with antibiotic changes made in 11% of patients. Regimen changes for nonresponders were empiric rather than based on microbiologic studies in 85% of cases. No mortality difference was observed between nonresponders in whom antibiotics were changed empirically versus based on microbiologic studies, suggesting that microbiologic studies have little influence on both treatment decisions and outcomes. The study was limited by exclusion of certain patients (e.g., HIV/AIDS, bronchiectasis, and recent hospitalization) more likely to be infected with unusual and resistant organisms.

To prospectively evaluate consensus recommendations to initially treat CAP with empiric antibiotics, a 2005 trial randomized 262 hospitalized adults (>18 years) to pathogen-directed treatment versus ATS guideline–driven empiric antibiotic treatment.[7] When microbiologic studies did not definitively reveal a culprit organism for patients in the

---

[6]Sanyal S, et al. Initial microbiologic studies did not affect outcome in adults hospitalized with community-acquired pneumonia. *Am J Respir Crit Care Med*. 1999;160(1):346-348.

[7]Van der Eerden MM, et al. Comparison between pathogen directed antibiotic treatment and empirical broad spectrum antibiotic treatment in patients with community acquired pneumonia: a prospective randomised study. *Thorax*. 2005;60(8):672-678.

pathogen-directed group, antibiotic selection was based on the suspected pathogen from the clinical presentation. Patients were included if their clinical presentations were suggestive of CAP (≥1 of the following: fever, dyspnea, chest pain, cough) and they had presence of new consolidation on CXR. Exclusion criteria included severe immunosuppression (e.g., immunosuppressive medications, HIV diagnosis), evidence of obstructive pneumonia or pneumonia after recent (<8 days) hospital discharge. The primary outcome was clinical efficacy, determined by length of stay (LOS). Secondary outcomes included 30-day mortality and clinical failure, which was defined as either early failure, in which signs and symptoms of pneumonia did not improve within 72 hours, or late failure, in which signs and symptoms returned after 72 hours.

There was no difference in the primary outcome (LOS of 14.3 vs. 13.2 days; P = .75), 30-day mortality (8% vs. 15%; P = .07), or clinical failure (21% vs. 23%; P = .66) between the pathogen-directed treatment and empiric antibiotic treatment groups. Notably, the study was powered for LOS, which can be influenced by factors unrelated to pneumonia, rather than mortality. Additionally, groups were imbalanced with respect to age (mean age 62 years in pathogen-directed group and 66.7 years in empiric treatment group; P = .03).

These studies suggest that empiric therapy based on ATS guidelines is a reasonable treatment strategy for those with CAP. This approach is consistent with IDSA guidelines,[3] which recommend empiric antibiotic treatment for most patients with CAP (moderate recommendation; level I evidence).

> After 48 hours of hospitalization, the patient remains afebrile and hemodynamically stable with HR in the 80s and SBP in the 120s. You consider whether it would be appropriate to transition him to an oral antibiotic.

When should hospitalized patients with CAP be transitioned to oral antibiotics?

Patients should be transitioned from IV to oral antibiotic therapy as soon as they are clinically stable.

A 2001 multicenter, randomized controlled trial examined two facets of inpatient antibiotic therapy: the efficacy of oral antibiotics as initial treatment for patients with nonsevere pneumonia and the efficacy of an early switch from IV to oral treatment in patients with severe pneumonia.[8] In this study, 85 hospitalized patients with nonsevere CAP were randomized to either oral antibiotics from admission or IV antibiotics with a switch to oral therapy once they had been afebrile for 72 hours. In an additional arm of the study, 103 patients with severe CAP initially treated with IV antibiotics were randomized to either an early switch to oral therapy at 48 hours or to completion of a full 10-day course of IV antibiotics. Severe CAP was defined as ≥1 criteria based upon a combination of the modified ATS minor criteria and the vital sign abnormalities included in the PSI. Patients requiring ICU level of care were excluded. Study outcomes included mortality, time to resolution of morbidity (the number of treatment days needed to achieve normalization of vital signs), and treatment failure (defined as clinical worsening requiring ICU admission, worsening after 2 days of appropriate treatment, or need to change the route of antibiotic administration).

Among patients with nonsevere CAP, there were no significant differences in mortality (0% vs. 2%, P = .3) or time to resolution of morbidity (≤5 days in 83% vs. 88%; P = .5) between oral and IV antibiotic therapy, respectively. Similarly, among patients with severe CAP, there were no differences in mortality (2% vs. 0%; P = .5), time to resolution of morbidity (≤5 days in 83% vs. 83%; P = .3), or treatment failure (25% vs. 24%; P = .9) between the early switch and no switch groups. However, the early switch group exhibited lower cost of treatment (P < .001) and length of hospitalization (6 vs. 11 days; P < .001).

A subsequent 2006 multicenter, randomized control trial assessed the effectiveness of an early switch to oral antibiotics in hospitalized patients with severe CAP.[9] In this trial, 265 patients with severe CAP, not requiring ICU admission, were randomized either to the intervention group, in which clinically stable patients were switched from IV to oral antibiotics after 72 hours to complete a total 10-day course of antibiotics, or to the control group, in which they received a total of 7 days of IV antibiotics. There was no significant difference in mortality at 28 days between the two groups, 4% for patients treated with IV to oral switch and 6% for patients treated with IV antibiotics for the entire duration (mean difference 2%, 95% CI −3 to 8%; no P-value reported).

---

[8]Castro-Guardiola A, et al. Efficacy and safety of oral and early-switch therapy for community-acquired pneumonia: a randomized controlled trial. *Am J Med.* 2001;111(5):367-374.

[9]Oosterheert JJ, et al. Effectiveness of early switch from intravenous to oral antibiotics in severe community acquired pneumonia: multicentre randomised trial. *Br Med J.* 2006;333(7580):1193-1195.

Clinical cure, evaluated using preset discharge criteria, was 83% in the intervention group versus 85% in the control (mean difference 2%, 95% CI −7 to 10%; no P-value reported). LOS was significantly shorter in the intervention group at 9.6 compared to 11.5 days in the control group (mean difference 1.9 days, 95% CI 0.6-3.2 days; no P-value reported).

These studies are consistent with IDSA guidelines in suggesting that many patients with CAP can transition from IV to oral antibiotics after achieving clinical stability, typically between 48 to 72 hours after initiating treatment (strong recommendation; level II evidence).[3]

> The patient remains clinically stable and discharges home on hospital day 3, with a plan to complete a 5-day course of oral amoxicillin and azithromycin for CAP.

KEY LEARNING POINTS

1. Patients who may be suitable for outpatient treatment can be identified using severity of illness scores and prognostic models, such as the PSI and CURB-65.
2. In addition to patients requiring vasopressors and/or mechanical ventilation, direct ICU admission is recommended for patients with ≥3 IDSA/ATS minor criteria for severe CAP.
3. There is no mortality difference between pathogen-directed therapy and empiric therapy in patients with CAP.
4. Patients should be transitioned from IV to oral antibiotic therapy as soon as they are clinically stable.

HEART FAILURE EXACERBATION

Megan U. Roosen-Runge, MD, MPH,
Shobha W. Stack, MD, PhD

You admit a 62-year-old woman presenting with dyspnea, whose examination is notable for oxygen saturation of 88% on ambient air, diffuse end-expiratory wheezes, and bilateral rales. While you suspect a chronic obstructive pulmonary disease (COPD) exacerbation, you want to ensure you are not overlooking heart failure (HF) exacerbation as the cause of her symptoms.

What is the utility of natriuretic peptides in differentiating HF exacerbation from other causes of dyspnea?

Natriuretic peptide levels are valuable in ruling out HF exacerbation as a cause of dyspnea, though results must be considered in the context of obesity, renal dysfunction, and angiotensin receptor neprilysin inhibitor (ARNI) use.

Breathing Not Properly[1] was a multicenter prospective study that demonstrated the value of B-type natriuretic peptide (BNP) levels among 1586 patients presenting to the ED with acute dyspnea. The diagnosis of HF exacerbation was made clinically by ED physicians and confirmed by two cardiologists who had access to medical records but were blinded to BNP levels. Compared to diagnostic criteria based on history, physical examination findings, or other

---

[1]Maisel AS, et al. Rapid measurement of B-type natriuretic peptide in the emergency diagnosis of heart failure. *N Engl J Med.* 2002;346:161-167.

laboratory tests, BNP was more able to identify (accuracy of 83.4% at a cut-off of ≥100 pg/mL) and rule out HF exacerbation as the cause of dyspnea (negative predictive value of 96% at a cut-off of <50 pg/mL, 95% CI 94%-97%).

A 2015 meta-analysis, which included Breathing Not Properly, provided additional evidence about the diagnostic utility of BNP and of N-terminal pro B-type natriuretic peptide (NT-proBNP, a biologically inactive prohormone that becomes active BNP when its N-terminal fragment is cleaved) in patients presenting to acute care with dyspnea.[2] Based on 15,263 natriuretic peptide test results, lower thresholds (BNP <100 pg/mL, NT-proBNP <300 pg/mL) have high sensitivity (95% and 99%, respectively), high negative predictive value (94% and 98%, respectively), but low specificity (67% and 43%, respectively) for diagnosing HF exacerbation. There was no statistically significant difference in diagnostic accuracy between BNP and NT-proBNP. These findings support the use of BNPs in ruling out HF exacerbation as a cause of acute dyspnea.

A 2015 meta-analysis investigated the diagnostic accuracy of NT-proBNP for ruling out HF exacerbation in patients with chronic kidney disease,[3] suggesting that higher cutoff values should be used in this setting. Because BNP is metabolized by adipose tissue, levels may be inappropriately low in obese patients with an elevated body mass index.[4] Because BNP is a substrate for neprilysin, use of an ARNI will increase BNP levels, such that a rising BNP level could reflect treatment response, exacerbation, and/or treatment failure.[5] These findings suggest that BNP levels should be interpreted in view of renal dysfunction, obesity, and ARNI use.

---

[2]Roberts E, et al. The diagnostic accuracy of the natriuretic peptides in heart failure: systematic review and diagnostic meta-analysis in the acute care setting. *Br Med J*. 2015;350(h910): 1-16.

[3]Schaub JA, et al. Amino-terminal pro B-type natriuretic peptide for diagnosis and prognosis in patients with renal dysfunction: a systematic review and meta-analysis. *JACC Heart Fail*. 2015;3(12):977-989.

[4]Madamanchi C, et al. Obesity and natriuretic peptides, BNP and NT-proBNP: mechanisms and diagnostic implications for heart failure. *Int J Cardiol*. 2014;176:611-617.

[5]Clerico A, et al. New issues on measurement of B-type natriuretic peptide. *Clin Chem Lab Med*. 2018;56(1):32-39.

Your patient has a normal BNP and is admitted for COPD exacerbation.

You evaluate another new admission, a 53-year-old woman with chronic HF with reduced ejection fraction (HFrEF) and left ventricular ejection fraction (LVEF) of 35%, who presents with mild tachypnea, hypoxemia, and tachycardia. Her chest radiograph demonstrates the following:

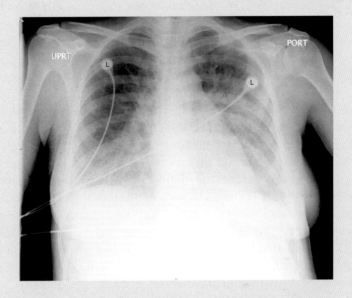

Based on her symptoms, elevated BNP, imaging findings, and 8 kg of weight gain, you diagnose the patient with a HF exacerbation and plan to diurese her with intravenous furosemide.

What is the preferred way to administer intravenous furosemide in HF exacerbations?

Outcomes are comparable between bolus and continuous intravenous furosemide dosing, with high doses associated with greater initial weight and fluid loss without long-term effect on renal function. Patients on high outpatient doses may benefit more from bolus than continuous administration.

DOSE-AHF[6] was a multinational, double-blind, randomized controlled trial assessing intravenous furosemide dosing in HF exacerbation. In a factorial design, 308 patients were randomized to continuous infusion versus twice daily bolus dosing, as well as low-dose (equivalent to the outpatient oral dose) versus high-dose (2.5 times the outpatient oral dose) furosemide. Patients were eligible to participate if they had presented to the hospital within the prior 24 hours with at least one sign and one symptom of HF exacerbation and had received an oral loop diuretic (furosemide 80-240 mg daily or equivalent dose) for at least 1 month prior to hospitalization. Patients were excluded for signs of cardiogenic shock such as systolic blood pressure <90 mm Hg, serum Cr >3 mg/dL, or requirement of vasodilators or inotropic agents other than digoxin. Primary outcomes included symptomatic improvement (assessed via patients' global assessment of symptoms quantified via the area under the curve) and increase in creatinine (from baseline to 72 hours). Secondary outcomes included net fluid loss.

There was no significant difference between continuous and bolus dosing in terms of symptomatic improvement ($P = .47$) or Cr increase (mean change 0.05 + 0.3 mg/dL with bolus dosing vs. 0.07 + 0.3 mg/dL with continuous infusion; $P = .45$). There was greater net fluid loss at 72 hours in the high-dose group (4899 + 3479 mL vs. 3575 + 2635 mL; $P = .001$). Compared to low-dose group, the high-dose group also had a greater proportion of patients who had a >0.3 mg/dL Cr increase at 72 hours (23% vs. 14%; $P = .04$) but not at 60 days ($P > .05$).

To evaluate whether these results were a function of outpatient furosemide dose prior to hospitalization, a follow-up analysis of DOSE-AHF compared bolus versus continuous intravenous furosemide administration and stratified outcomes by higher (≥120 mg/d) versus lower (<120 mg/d) outpatient furosemide equivalent doses.[7] Multivariate regression analysis revealed that for every 10 mg more of outpatient furosemide equivalent dose, bolus administration was associated with more net fluid loss at 72 hours (95 mL more vs. 88 mL less in the continuous infusion group, $P = .02$).

A meta-analysis of 10 randomized clinical trials (including DOSE-AHF) comparing continuous and bolus administration among 518 total

---

[6]Felker GM, et al. Diuretic strategies in patients with acute decompensated heart failure. *N Engl J Med*. 2011;364(9):797-805.

[7]Shah RV, et al. Effect of admission oral diuretic dose on response to continuous versus bolus intravenous diuretics in acute heart failure: an analysis from diuretic optimization strategies in acute heart failure. *Am Heart J*. 2012;164(6):862-868.

patients found no difference in the incidence of increased creatinine (weighted mean difference [WMD] 0, 95% CI −0.09 to 0.09; $P = .31$), length of hospitalization (WMD −1.06, 95% CI −3.88 to 1.76; $P = .06$), or all-cause mortality (RR 1.13, 95% CI 0.61-2.10; $P = .49$).[8] The difference in weight loss significantly favored continuous infusion (WMD 0.78 kg, 95% CI 0.03-1.54; $P = .04$).

You start the patient on bolus dose furosemide. While completing her medication reconciliation, you notice metoprolol on her home medication list and consider whether to continue this during her hospital stay.

When treating patients with HF exacerbations, when should beta-blockers be continued?

Among patients not requiring dobutamine support, beta-blocker continuation during HF exacerbation is noninferior to discontinuation.

The B-CONVINCED trial[9] was a randomized controlled noninferiority study conducted at 28 sites among 169 patients with HF exacerbation previously on stable beta-blocker therapy who were randomized to continuation versus discontinuation of beta-blockade. Patients with more severe exacerbations (i.e., need for dobutamine support) were excluded. The primary outcome was the physician-evaluated symptomatic improvement (percentage of patients with improvement in general wellbeing and dyspnea at 3 days based on physician assessment). Secondary outcomes included patient-reported symptomatic improvement (percentage of patients with self-reported improvement in general wellbeing and dyspnea at day 3), hospital length of stay, rate of rehospitalization at 3 months, rate of death at 3 months, and the proportion of patients receiving a beta-blocker at 3 months.

There was no between-group difference in the primary outcome (92.8% vs. 92.3%, unilateral 95% CI −7.6% to 6.6% with upper limit below predefined noninferiority limit of 12.5%; no P-value reported). Beta-blocker continuation was noninferior to discontinuation in terms

---

[8] Wu MY, et al. Loop diuretic strategies in patients with acute decompensated heart failure: a meta-analysis of randomized controlled trials. *J Crit Care*. 2014;29(1):2-9.

[9] Jondeau G, et al. B-CONVINCED: Beta-blocker CONtinuation Vs. INterruption in patients with Congestive heart failure hospitalizED for a decompensation episode. *Eur Heart J*. 2009;30(18):2186-2192.

of patient-reported symptomatic improvement (88.4% vs. 82.7%, upper limit of unilateral 95% CI 3.8%), hospital length of stay (11.5 + 8.3 days vs. 10.4 + 9.7 days; P = .2), and mortality rate at 3 months (9% vs. 8%; P = .83). Notably, the number of patients taking beta-blockers at 3 months was significantly higher in the continuation versus discontinuation group (90% vs. 76%, P = .04). Evidence of benefits from continuation in the inpatient setting is consistent with European Society of Cardiology (ESC) guidelines about well-established benefits of chronic therapy in the outpatient setting (level A, class I).[10]

> You continue her metoprolol. The patient's dyspnea resolves after 3 days, and she returns to her dry weight. However, she is still functionally limited by HF symptoms. You want to ensure that she is on optimal medical therapy (OMT) as she transitions back to the outpatient setting.

What is OMT for patients with chronic HFrEF?

In many patients, OMT consists of a beta-blocker, aldosterone antagonist, and either an angiotensin-converting enzyme inhibitor (ACE-I), angiotensin receptor blocker (ARB), ARNI, or ivabradine. Hydralazine and isosorbide dinitrate should also be considered in symptomatic black patients.

A series of trials have demonstrated that beta-blockers confer a mortality benefit in HF patients. MERIT-HF was a 1999 randomized control trial to demonstrate a mortality reduction with the use of metoprolol CR/XL versus placebo in patients with symptomatic HFrEF (RR 0.66, 95% CI 0.53-0.81).[11] These findings were bolstered by the CIBIS-II[12] and COPERNICUS[13] trials, which found mortality benefits

---

[10]Dickstein K, et al. ESC guidelines for the diagnosis and treatment of acute and chronic heart failure 2008: the task force for the diagnosis and treatment of acute and chronic heart failure 2008 of the European Society of Cardiology. Developed in collaboration with the Heart Failure Association of the ESC (HFA) and endorsed by the European Society of Intensive Care Medicine (ESICM). *Eur Heart J.* 2008;29:2388-2442.

[11]Fagerberg B, et al. Effect of metoprolol CR/XL in chronic heart failure: Metoprolol CR/XL randomised intervention trial in congestive heart failure. *Lancet.* 1999;353(9169):2001-2007.

[12]CIBIS Authors. The Cardiac Insufficiency Bisoprolol Study II (CIBIS-II): a randomised trial. *Lancet.* 1999;353(9146):9-13.

[13]Packer M, et al. Effect of Carvedilol on the morbidity of patients with severe chronic heart failure. *Circulation.* 2002;106(17):2194-2199.

with bisoprolol and carvedilol, respectively. Together, these studies led to guidelines that recommend the use of beta-blockers in all patients with HFrEF (level C, class I).[14]

Several randomized controlled trials established the role of aldosterone antagonists in chronic HFrEF. In RALES, 1663 patients were randomized to receive daily spironolactone or placebo.[15] Inclusion criteria were New York Heart Association (NYHA) class IV HF in the 6 months prior to enrollment, HFrEF, LVEF<35%, and current NYHA class III-IV symptoms despite therapy with an ACE-I (if tolerated) and a loop diuretic. Exclusion criteria included operable valvular heart disease, serum creatinine >2.5 mg/dL, and serum potassium >5.0 mEq/L. Based on the 30% reduction in all-cause mortality observed in the spironolactone group (RR 0.70, 95% CI 0.60-0.82, $P < .001$) and similar conclusions from subsequent studies,[16,17] the American College of Cardiology Foundation (ACCF)/American Heart Association (AHA) guidelines recommend aldosterone antagonists as part of goal-direct medical therapy for patients with ≤% and NYHA class II-IV in the absence of contraindications (level A, class I).[18]

The role of ACE-Is in HF was established in CONSENSUS,[19] a trial that demonstrated a reduction in 6-month mortality among 253 patients with NYHA class IV HFrEF taking enalapril in addition to standard medical therapy versus placebo (26% vs. 44%, $P = .002$). Similarly, the role of ARBs was demonstrated in the CHARM-Alternative trial,[20] in which 2028 patients with NYHA class II-IV HFrEF who were intolerant of ACE-Is were randomized to candesartan versus placebo in addition to standard medical therapy. At a median follow-up of 33.7 months,

---

[14]Yancy CW, et al. 2013 ACCF/AHA guideline for the management of heart failure. *Circulation.* 2013;128:e240-e327.

[15]Pitt B, et al. The effect of spironolactone on morbidity and mortality in patients with severe heart failure. *N Engl J Med.* 1999;341(10):709-717.

[16]Zannad F, et al. Eplerenone in patients with systolic heart failure and mild symptoms. *N Engl J Med.* 2011;364:11-21.

[17]Pitt B, et al. Eplerenone, a selective aldosterone blocker, in patients with left ventricular dysfunction after myocardial infarction. *N Engl J Med.* 2003;348:1309-1321.

[18]Yancy CW, et al. 2013 ACCF/AHA guideline for the management of heart failure. *J Am Coll Cardiol.* 2013;62(16):e147-e239.

[19]CONSENSUS Trial Study Group. Effects of enalapril on mortality in severe congestive heart failure, results of the cooperative north Scandinavian enalapril survival study. *N Engl J Med.* 1987;316(23):1429-1435.

[20]Granger CB, et al. Effects of candesartan in patients with chronic heart failure and reduced left-ventricular systolic function intolerant to angiotensin-converting-enzyme inhibitors: the CHARM-Alternative trial. *Lancet.* 2003;362(9386):772-776.

fewer patients receiving candesartan experienced the composite of cardiovascular death or HF admission (HR 0.70, 95% CI 0.60-0.81, $P < .001$).

PARADIGM-HF[21] was a 2014 randomized, double-blind trial among 914 patients with NYHA class II-IV symptoms that demonstrated treatment with an ANRI-reduced cardiovascular mortality (13.3% vs. 16.5%, $P < .001$) and first hospitalization for HF exacerbation (12.8% vs. 15.6%, $P < .001$) compared to enalapril alone. The 2016 American College of Cardiology (ACC)/AHA/Heart Failure Society of America (HFSA) guidelines recommend that patients with NYHA class II-III HFrEF who tolerate an ACE-I or ARB be switched to ARNI (level B-R, class I).[22]

The role of ivabradine in chronic HFrEF was evaluated in SHIFT,[23] a multicenter placebo-controlled study that randomized 6558 patients in sinus rhythm (HR $\geq$ 70 bpm) to ivabradine versus placebo in addition to other HF therapies. Ivabradine was associated with a lower primary composite outcome of cardiovascular death or HF hospitalization (HR 0.82, 95% CI 0.75-0.90; $P < .001$), resulting in its inclusion in 2017 ACCF/AHA HF guidelines[24] (level B-R, class IIa).

A-HeFT, a multicenter randomized, doubled-blind, placebo-controlled trial,[25] evaluated the effect of isosorbide dinitrate plus hydralazine among 1050 patients with NYHA class III-IV HFrEF who self-identified as black. Compared to placebo, isosorbide dinitrate plus hydralazine reduced a weighted primary composite outcome reflecting all-cause mortality, first HF hospitalization, and change in quality of life (HR 0.57, $P = .01$). Secondary outcomes of and first HF hospitalization were both lower among patients receiving isosorbide dinitrate plus hydralazine also had lower all-cause mortality (6.2 vs. 10.2%, $P = .02$, number needed to treat [NNT] = 25) and first HF hospitalization (16.4% vs. 24.4%, $P = .001$, NNT = 13), prompting early trial

---

[21]McMurray JJV, et al. Angiotensin-neprilysin inhibition versus enalapril in heart failure. *N Engl J Med.* 2014;371(11):993-1004.

[22]Yancy CW, et al. 2016 ACC/AHA/HFSA focused update on new pharmacological therapy for heart failure: an update of the 2013 ACCF/AHA guideline for the management of heart failure. *Circulation.* 2016;134:e282-e293.

[23]Swedberg K, et al. Ivabradine and outcomes in chronic heart failure (SHIFT): a randomised placebo-controlled study. *Lancet.* 2010;376(10):875-885.

[24]Yancy CW, et al. 2017 ACC/AHA/HFSA focused update of the 2013 ACCF/AHA guideline for the management of heart failure. *J Am Coll Cardiol.* 2017;70(6):776-803.

[25]Taylor AL, et al. Combination of isosorbide dinitrate and hydralazine in blacks with heart failure. *N Engl J Med.* 2004;351:2049-2057.

termination. The ACCF/AHA HF guidelines[18] support consideration of hydralazine/isosorbide dinitrate among African American patients with persistent NYHA class III-IV symptoms (level A, class I).

> The patient has NYHA class III symptoms at baseline. Her outpatient medications include lisinopril, metoprolol, spironolactone, and furosemide. You discharge her with a recommendation to follow-up and discuss with her cardiologist about replacing lisinopril with sacubitril-valsartan.

KEY LEARNING POINTS

1. Natriuretic peptide levels are valuable in ruling out HF exacerbation as a cause of dyspnea, though results must be considered in the context of obesity, renal dysfunction, and ARNI use.
2. Outcomes are comparable between bolus and continuous intravenous furosemide dosing in HF exacerbation, with high doses associated with greater initial weight and fluid loss without long-term effect on renal function. Patients on high outpatient doses may benefit more from bolus than continuous administration.
3. Among patients not requiring dobutamine support, beta-blocker continuation during HF exacerbation is noninferior to discontinuation.
4. In many patients, OMT consists of a beta-blocker, aldosterone antagonist, and either an ACE-I, ARB, ARNI, or ivabradine. Hydralazine and isosorbide dinitrate should also be considered in symptomatic black patients.

ATRIAL FIBRILLATION

Michael Charles C. Tan, MD,
Kristen M. Rogers, MD, MPH

You admit a 67-year-old woman with a history of hypertension and diabetes from the ED with several days of new, subacute shortness of breath and palpitations. Besides a heart rate in the 150s, her vitals are normal. Cardiopulmonary examination reveals an irregularly irregular heartbeat without murmurs, jugular venous distension, lower extremity edema, or crackles. She denies syncope, orthopnea, paroxysmal nocturnal dyspnea, or exertional dyspnea. Her ECG demonstrates the following (Figure 16.1):

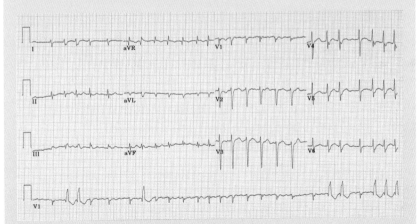

Figure 16.1 This ECG demonstrates a narrow complex, irregularly irregular tachycardia with intermittent premature ventricular contractions. (Reprinted from Rimmerman CM. *Interactive Electrocardiography*. Philadelphia: Wolters Kluwer; 2016, with permission.)

(continued)

You diagnose her with atrial fibrillation (AF) with rapid ventricular response and decide to treat her with an IV beta-blocker. With this treatment, her HR subsequently decreases to 105 to 110 bpm, and her symptoms resolve. Repeat ECG after this improvement demonstrates the following (Figure 16.2):

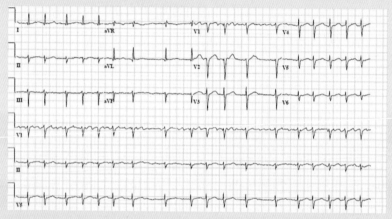

Figure 16.2 This ECG shows an irregularly irregular rhythm, now with decreased ventricular rate. (Reprinted from Herzog E. *The Cardiac Care Unit Survival Guide.* Philadelphia: Wolters Kluwer; 2012, with permission.)

A transthoracic echocardiogram shows normal left ventricular and valvular function. You would like to transition her to an oral medication for her AF.

What is the role of rate or rhythm control in the long-term pharmacologic treatment of patients with nonvalvular AF?

In patients with nonvalvular AF without preexcitation or heart failure, rate and rhythm control strategies are associated with similar mortality and quality of life. Rhythm control is associated with more frequent adverse events, though it may be appropriate in certain clinical scenarios (e.g., symptomatic patients, those unable to achieve rate control).

This question was studied in AFFIRM,[1] a multicenter, parallel-group, randomized control trial of 4060 patients with nonvalvular AF.

---

[1]The Atrial Fibrillation Follow-up Investigation of Rhythm Management (AFFIRM) Investigators. A comparison of rate control and rhythm control in patients with atrial fibrillation. *N Engl J Med.* 2002;347(23):1825-1833.

Participants were ≥65 years old and felt to have recurrent AF, risk factors for stroke or death, and need for long-term anticoagulation. Individuals were excluded for contraindications to anticoagulation or inability to tolerate ≥two medications in either treatment strategy. AFFIRM randomized individuals to either a rate or rhythm control strategy. In the rate control group, drugs such as beta-blockers, calcium-channel blockers, or digoxin were used to target heart rates of ≤80 bpm at rest and ≤110 bpm with activity (measured via 6-minute walk test or 24-hr ambulatory ECG). In the rhythm control group, class Ia, Ic, or III antiarrhythmic agents, along with electrical cardioversion, were used to achieve and maintain sinus rhythm. All patients were anticoagulated with warfarin (goal INR 2-3), though at the discretion of their physicians, individuals in the rhythm control group who maintained normal sinus rhythm for ≥4 weeks could discontinue anticoagulation. Individuals in either arm who failed pharmacologic treatment could consider radio-frequency ablation, maze procedure, or pacing techniques. The primary outcome was all-cause mortality. The secondary outcome was a composite of death, disability, stroke, anoxic encephalopathy, major bleeding, and cardiac arrest.

There was no difference between rate and rhythm control strategies in the primary (25.9% vs. 26.7%, HR 1.15, 95% CI 0.99-1.34; $P = .08$) or secondary ($P = .33$) outcomes. A subgroup analysis showed that rhythm control was associated with increased risk of death in patients ≥65 years old, with coronary artery disease (CAD), and without heart failure. Rate control was not associated with increased adverse events; notable adverse events in the rhythm control group included increased hospitalization rates ($P < .001$) and torsade de pointes ($P = .007$). Caveats include limited generalizability to younger patients and those without stroke risk factors, as well as the exclusion of patients with frequent or severe symptoms deemed unsuitable for rate control.

The 2014 American Heart Association (AHA)/American College of Cardiology (ACC) guidelines[2] recommend a rate control strategy with a beta-blocker or nondihydropyridine calcium-channel blocker for individuals with paroxysmal, persistent, or permanent AF (class I, level B). Rhythm control remains appropriate for patients who are unable to achieve rate control or who remain symptomatic despite rate control. Additionally, because conversion and maintenance of sinus rhythm is more difficult in individuals who remain in AF, some patients—such as

---

[2]January CT, et al. 2014 AHA/ACC/HRS guideline for the management of patients with atrial fibrillation: executive summary: a report of the American College of Cardiology/American Heart Association Task Force on practice guidelines and the Heart Rhythm Society. *Circulation.* 2014;130(23):2071-104.

those who are younger or whose cardiac output is significantly impaired by arrhythmias—may benefit from restoration of sinus rhythm.

You start the patient on an oral beta-blocker, with good rate control and resolution of symptoms. During medication counseling, you discuss her target heart rate. She wonders how fast is "too fast."

What is a reasonable heart rate target in chronic rate control of AF?

A lenient heart rate target of <110 bpm at rest is associated with similar outcomes as a strict target of <80 bpm and is a reasonable target for management of asymptomatic permanent AF in patients with preserved left ventricular (LV) systolic function.

RACE-II[3] was a prospective, multicenter, open-label, parallel-group, randomized controlled noninferiority trial that compared lenient versus strict HR control in 614 patients with permanent AF. Participants were ≤80 years old, had a mean resting HR > 80 bpm, and were on either oral anticoagulation or aspirin based on thromboembolic risk factors. Participants were randomized to lenient-control with a target resting HR < 110 bpm versus strict-control with target resting HR < 80 bpm and <110 bpm with moderate exercise. Rate control was achieved with beta-blockers, nondihydropyridine calcium-channel blockers, and digoxin, alone or in combination. The primary outcome was a composite of cardiovascular death, heart failure, hospitalization, stroke, systemic embolism, bleeding, and clinically significant arrhythmic events. Secondary outcomes were components of the primary outcome, along with all-cause mortality, and AF symptoms (e.g., dyspnea, fatigue, palpitations, functional status based on New York Heart Association (NYHA) classification).

After median follow-up of 3 years, there was no difference in the primary outcome (12.9% in lenient-control group vs. 14.9% in the strict-control group, HR 0.84, 90% CI 0.58-1.21; $P < .001$ for the prespecified noninferiority margin) or secondary outcomes. Caveats include exclusion of patients with history of stroke, resulting in a relatively low-risk study population, and between-group variation in achieving HR targets (67% among strict-control vs. 98% among lenient-control). Given these findings, the AHA/ACC guidelines[2] recommend that lenient rate–control with a target resting HR of <110 bpm is appropriate for

---

[3]Van Gelder IC, et al. Lenient versus strict rate control in patients with atrial fibrillation. *N Engl J Med.* 2010;362(15):1363-1373.

asymptomatic individuals with AF who have a preserved ejection fraction (class IIb, level B). For individuals who are symptomatic at these HRs, a resting HR of <80 bpm should be targeted (class IIa, level B).

The patient asks about what options exist to "cure" her abnormal heart rhythm. You mention direct-current cardioversion (DCCV) as one way to restore normal sinus rhythm, and she asks what that would entail.

What are potential strategies for using elective DCCV to achieve rhythm control in patients with AF?

Transesophageal echocardiogram (TEE)-guided DCCV is a reasonable alternative to a conventional strategy of delayed DCCV (after 3 weeks of therapeutic anticoagulation) for some patients.

ACUTE[4]—a multicenter, prospective, randomized control trial—randomized 1222 individuals ≥18 years old with AF ≥2 days to TEE-guided DCCV with short-term anticoagulation versus conventional prolonged anticoagulation prior to DCCV. In the TEE-guided group, inpatients were therapeutically anticoagulated with IV unfractionated heparin for 24 hours and then underwent TEE to assess for thrombi in the left atrial appendage. If no clot was visualized, DCCV was attempted. Outpatients received TEE-guided DCCV after 5 days of having achieved therapeutic anticoagulation with warfarin (goal INR 2-3). In the conventional therapy group, patients were empirically anticoagulated with warfarin for 3 weeks prior to DCCV. In both groups, patients were anticoagulated for 4 weeks after cardioversion. Exclusion criteria included history of atrial flutter without AF, hemodynamic instability, and long-term anticoagulation (≥7 days). The primary outcome was the composite rate of cerebrovascular accident, transient ischemic attack, and peripheral embolism. Secondary outcomes included hemorrhagic events, death, return to and maintenance of sinus rhythm, and functional status.

The primary outcome did not differ by treatment group (0.8% vs. 0.5%, RR = 1.62; P = .50). Hemorrhagic events were less frequent in the TEE-guided group (2.9% vs. 5.5%, RR = 0.53; P = .03), but there were no differences in death, immediate return to or maintenance of sinus

---

[4]Klein AL, et al. Use of transesophageal echocardiography to guide cardioversion in patients with atrial fibrillation. *N Engl J Med.* 2001;344(19):1411-1420.

rhythm, or functional status. Caveats include a lower-than-anticipated thromboembolism rate and greater difficulty maintaining therapeutic anticoagulation in the conventional group.

The AHA/ACC guidelines[2] note that compared to a conventional strategy, TEE-guided DCCV is a reasonable alternative for individuals with AF of ≥48 hours duration or of unknown duration who have not had 3 weeks of anticoagulation (class IIa, level B).

> Upon arrival to the medicine ward, the patient has heart rates in the 80 to 90s on scheduled oral beta-blockers. As you prepare her medication reconciliation list, you wonder if she could benefit from anticoagulation to reduce the risk of the cardioembolic complications from AF.

How can the risk of thromboembolic complications and appropriateness of anticoagulation be evaluated in patients with AF?

In nonvalvular AF, the CHA_2DS_2-VASc score can be used to identify patients at intermediate or high risk of embolic stroke (CHA_2DS_2-VASc score ≥2) who should be anticoagulated.

The $CHADS_2$ score[5] was created to address this issue by combining features of two existing classification schemes previously derived by the Atrial Fibrillation Investigators (AFI) and the Stroke Prevention in Atrial Fibrillation III (SPAF-III) group. When compared to its predecessors, the $CHADS_2$ score demonstrated the greatest ability to quantify stroke risk with a c-statistic of 0.82 (95% CI 80-84%) compared to 0.68 (95% CI 65%-71%) for AFI and 0.74 (95% CI 71%-76%) for SPAF-III.

Subsequently, the $CHADS_2$ score was further refined via the CHA_2DS_2-VASc score,[6] which was created to account for several additional risk factors and address concerns over the high proportion of individuals risk stratified into the "intermediate-risk" category ($CHADS_2 = 1$, 61.9% of individuals). In a real-world cohort of 1084 patients from the Euro Heart Survey for AF, CHA_2DS_2-VASc demonstrated a greater ability

---

[5]Gage BF, et al. Validation of clinical classification schemes for predicting stroke: results from the National Registry of Atrial Fibrillation. *J Am Med Assoc*. 2001;285(22):2864-2870.
[6]Lip GY, et al. Refining clinical risk stratification for predicting stroke and thromboembolism in atrial fibrillation using a novel risk factor-based approach: the euro heart survey on atrial fibrillation. *Chest*. 2010;137(2):263-272.

than $CHADS_2$ to stratify individuals across risk categories, categorizing fewer individuals as intermediate risk (15.1% versus 61.9%). Additionally, CHA_2DS_2-VASc performed better at identifying patients at low risk for embolic events (0% in the "low-risk" category with thromboembolism versus 1.4% among those identified as intermediate risk using $CHADS_2$).

Given the demonstrated efficacy of warfarin in risk reduction of embolic events, the AHA/ACC guidelines[2] recommend anticoagulation for individuals with nonvalvular AF and history of stroke, transient ischemic attack, or CHA_2DS_2-VASc score ≥ 2 (class I, level B).

CHA_2DS_2-VASc Scoring Algorithm	
Risk Factor	Score
Congestive heart failure (or LV dysfunction)	1
Hypertension (>140/90 or medically treated)	1
Age $\geq$ 75 years	2
Diabetes mellitus	1
History of stroke or, TIA, or thromboembolism	2
Vascular disease (e.g., peripheral artery disease, myocardial infarction, or aortic plaque)	1
Age 65-74	1
Sex category (female)	1

LV, left ventricular; TIA, transient ischemic attack.

(Reprinted from Lip GY, et al. Refining clinical risk stratification for predicting stroke and thromboembolism in atrial fibrillation using a novel risk factor-based approach: the euro heart survey on atrial fibrillation. *Chest.* 2010;137(2):263-272, with permission.)

The adjusted annual stroke rates for individuals provided below.

Stroke Risk Stratification for $CHADS_2$ and CHA_2DS_2-VASc Scores			
$CHADS_2$		CHA_2DS_2-VASc	
Score	Adjusted Stroke Rate (% per year)	Score	Adjusted Stroke Rate (% per year)
0	1.9%	0	0.0%
1	2.8%	1	1.3%
2	4.0%	2	2.2%
3	5.9%	3	3.2%

(continued)

Stroke Risk Stratification for CHADS$_2$ and CHA$_2$DS$_2$-VASc Scores			
CHADS$_2$		CHA$_2$DS$_2$-VASc	
Score	Adjusted Stroke Rate (% per year)	Score	Adjusted Stroke Rate (% per year)
4	8.5%	4	4.0%
5	12.5%	5	6.7%
6	18.2%	6	9.8%
–	–	7	9.6%
–	–	8	6.7%
–	–	9	15.2%

(**CHADS$_2$** data from Gage BF, et al. Validation of clinical classification schemes for predicting stroke: results from the National Registry of Atrial Fibrillation. *J Am Med Assoc.* 2001;285(22):2864-2870. **CHA$_2$DS$_2$-VASc** data from Lip GY, et al. Refining clinical risk stratification for predicting stroke and thromboembolism in atrial fibrillation using a novel risk factor-based approach: the euro heart survey on atrial fibrillation. *Chest.* 2010;137(2): 263-272.)

Your patient's CHA$_2$DS$_2$-VASc = 4 for hypertension, female gender, age 65 to 74, and diabetes. You recommend oral anticoagulation, to which the patient agrees. She remains stable and is discharged home on anticoagulation with plans to pursue DCCV in 3 weeks.

KEY LEARNING POINTS

1. In patients with nonvalvular AF without preexcitation or heart failure, rate and rhythm control strategies are associated with similar mortality and quality of life. Rhythm control is associated with more frequent adverse events, though it may be appropriate in certain clinical scenarios (e.g., symptomatic patients, those unable to achieve rate control).
2. A lenient heart rate target of <110 bpm at rest is associated with similar outcomes as a strict target of <80 bpm and is a reasonable target for management of asymptomatic permanent AF in patients with preserved LV systolic function.
3. TEE-guided DCCV is a reasonable alternative to a conventional strategy of delayed DCCV (after 3 weeks of therapeutic anticoagulation) for some patients.
4. In nonvalvular AF, the CHA$_2$DS$_2$-VASc score can be used to identify patients at intermediate or high risk of embolic stroke (CHA$_2$DS$_2$-VASc score ≥2) who should be anticoagulated.

CHRONIC OBSTRUCTIVE PULMONARY DISEASE EXACERBATION

Yilin Zhang, MD,
Jonathan Hourmozdi, MD

You are called by the ED to admit a 63-year-old man with severe chronic obstructive pulmonary disease (COPD) (FEV1 45%) and 3 days of progressive dyspnea and increased cough. While in the ED, he also coughs up a large amount of yellow-green sputum. You diagnose him with a COPD exacerbation and consider whether you should send a sputum culture.

What is the role of sputum culture in the evaluation of patients with COPD exacerbations?

A sputum culture does not need to be routinely sent in patients with COPD exacerbations but should be considered in patients with severe underlying disease or those hospitalized for COPD exacerbations with purulent sputum or requiring ventilatory support.

A 2007 prospective study[1] of 40 hospitalized patients compared sputum sample against bronchoscopic protected specimen brush (PSB), the gold standard for detecting distal airway infections, for isolation of bacterial pathogens in COPD exacerbations. All patients had a spirometric diagnosis of COPD and recent pulmonary function testing. Patients with pneumonia and recent antibiotic use were

---

[1]Soler N, et al. Bronchoscopic validation of the significance of sputum purulence in severe exacerbations of chronic obstructive pulmonary disease. *Thorax*. 2007;62:29-35.

excluded. Sputum samples and PSBs were collected within 24 hours of admission.

There was strong agreement between sputum and PSB culture results (κ = 0.85; P < .002). Patient-reported sputum purulence was strongly predictive of potentially pathogenic bacteria on PSB (OR 27.20, 95% CI 4.60-60.69; P = .001). Other predictive factors of PSB culture positivity were FEV1 <50% (OR 2.27, 95% CI 1.55-3.21; P = .01), >4 exacerbations in the past year (OR 6.91, 95% CI 1.24-38.52; P = .03), and hospitalization in the past 3 years (OR 4.13, 95% CI 1.02-16.67; P = .04). The overall sensitivity and specificity of sputum purulence for predicting PSB positivity were 89.5% and 76.5%, respectively. Generalizability is limited by the study's small size, inclusion of only men, and skew toward patients with more significant disease (the mean FEV1 of patients was 37% and >50% of patients reported >4 exacerbations per year). Additionally, while bronchoscopy is the gold standard for diagnosis of pneumonia, the authors used a threshold of $\geq 10^2$ cfu/mL, which is lower than the accepted threshold for bacterial infection[2,3] and may not adequately distinguish between colonization and infection.

Current guidelines recommend sputum analysis for patients with a COPD exacerbation and high likelihood of bacterial infection.[4,5] The 2018 Global Initiative for Chronic Obstructive Lung Disease (GOLD) guidelines recommend cultures in patients with frequent exacerbations, severe airflow limitation, or exacerbations requiring mechanical ventilation. The 2010 National Institute for Health and Clinical Excellence (NICE) guidelines recommend sputum microscopy and culture in all hospitalized patients with purulent sputum (grade D, based on expert opinion).

[2]Cabello H, et al. Bacterial colonization of distal airways in healthy subjects and chronic lung disease: a bronchoscopic study. *Eur Respir J.* 1997;10:1137-1144.

[3]Rosell A, et al. Microbiologic determinants of exacerbation in chronic obstructive pulmonary disease. *Arch Intern Med.* 2005;165:891-897.

[4]Global Initiative for Chronic Obstructive Lung Diseases. Global strategy for the diagnosis, management and prevention of chronic obstructive pulmonary disease (2018 report). *Global Initiative for Chronic Lung Disease, Inc.* 2018.

[5]National Institute for Health and Clinical Excellence. Chronic obstructive pulmonary disease: management of chronic pulmonary obstructive disease in adults in the primary and secondary care (partial update). London, National Clinical Guideline Center, 2010.

You discover that this is the patient's third hospitalization for COPD exacerbation this year. Based on his history of frequent exacerbations, severe obstruction, and sputum purulence, you decide to send his sputum for stain and culture. He denies any recent fevers or chills, and his chest radiograph demonstrates the following:

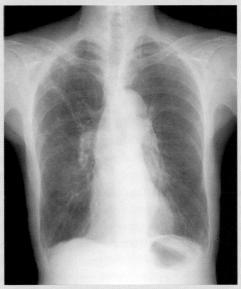

You do not observe any focal infiltrates. The nurse asks if you would like to start antibiotics while you await the sputum test results.

Should patients presenting to the hospital with COPD exacerbation routinely receive antibiotic therapy?

Antibiotics should be given to all patients requiring ventilatory support as well as those with sputum purulence and at least one additional cardinal symptom of COPD exacerbation.

Older studies of largely chronic bronchitis patients demonstrated that those with three cardinal symptoms of COPD exacerbation—increased sputum volume, sputum purulence, and dyspnea—benefited from antibiotics, in contrast to those with only one symptom.[4,6]

[6]Vollenweider DJ, et al. Antibiotics for exacerbations of chronic obstructive pulmonary disease. *Cochrane Database Syst Rev.* 2012;12:CD010257.

However, concerns about antibiotic resistance and adverse effects have compelled closer inspection of routine antibiotic use.

A meta-analysis reviewed 16 randomized controlled trials (RCTs) comparing antibiotics versus placebo in COPD exacerbations.[6] All trials included patients with a clinical or spirometric diagnosis of COPD and excluded patients with pneumonia. In treatment groups, antibiotics were administered for ≥2 days, with specific antibiotics including commonly used (e.g., amoxicillin-clavulanate, trimethoprim-sulfamethoxazole, doxycycline) and less common (e.g., chloramphenicol, tetracycline, streptomycin) agents. Notably, the most commonly used antibiotics, azithromycin and fluoroquinolones, were not studied in the trials included in this meta-analysis. The primary outcome was treatment failure through 4 weeks (defined as no resolution or deterioration of symptoms, death, or need for additional antibiotics during this period). Four trials exclusively evaluated patients hospitalized with COPD exacerbations on the wards and demonstrated that antibiotics reduced the risk of treatment failure up to 4 weeks (RR = 0.77, 95% CI 0.65-0.91; P = .002; number needed to treat [NNT] = 10). Secondary outcomes of all-cause mortality and length of stay did not differ significantly between antibiotic and placebo groups. In contrast, among ICU patients, antibiotics were associated with decreased mortality (Peto OR = 0.21, 95% CI 0.06-0.72; P = .01; NNT = 6) and length of stay (mean difference -9.60 days, 95% CI −12.84 to −6.36 days, P-value not reported).

A major caveat of this meta-analysis is that it did not routinely consider concurrent corticosteroid therapy, which is now accepted as standard of care. Other limitations include a broad definition of treatment failure, inclusion of studies in which patients received as few as 2 days of antibiotics (notably shorter than the standard treatment duration of 5-7 days), and poor generalizability to women, given a heavy skew toward men.

Because sputum purulence may be a marker of bacterial infection, the GOLD (level B, based on limited body of evidence or RCTs with important limitations) and NICE (grade A, based on evidence from systematic reviews or meta-analyses of RCTs) guidelines both recommend antibiotics in patients with increased sputum purulence.[4,5] The GOLD guidelines further specify that patients should have ≥1 additional cardinal symptom of COPD exacerbation including increased dyspnea or sputum production. Because of the mortality benefit in ICU patients, the GOLD guidelines also recommend antibiotics in patients with severe exacerbations that require either mechanical or noninvasive ventilatory support.

Because he has purulent sputum and increased dyspnea, you start the patient on levofloxacin along with inhaled albuterol and ipratropium. You admit him to the hospital and consider how to initiate treatment with systemic corticosteroids.

What is an appropriate initial approach for systemic corticosteroid therapy in COPD exacerbations?

Oral corticosteroids administered for 5 days at a dose equivalent to 40 mg of prednisone are an appropriate therapeutic regimen for patients with COPD exacerbations.

The optimal route of systemic steroids, a cornerstone of therapy for COPD exacerbation, was assessed in a secondary meta-analysis of three trials with 298 patients comparing oral versus IV corticosteroids.[7]

All patients had a spirometric diagnosis of obstruction and >10 pack-year smoking history. Patients with asthma were excluded. There was no significant difference in the primary outcomes of mortality, readmission, and treatment failure (defined as the need to intensify therapy through 5 months of follow-up). One trial showed an increased likelihood of hyperglycemia with IV steroids compared to oral steroids (55% vs. 20%, OR 4.89, 95% CI 1.20-19.94, P-value not reported), though this is confounded by the fact that patients in the IV group received higher doses of steroids.[8] This meta-analysis was limited by significant variability in dose and duration of corticosteroid treatments, which ranged from 7 days to several weeks, and the results were mainly driven by a large single-center European study.

Another meta-analysis of five trials with a total of 519 patients compared the efficacy of shorter (3-7 days) versus longer (10-15 days) treatment duration in COPD exacerbation.[9] Patients requiring ventilatory assistance were excluded. The main outcomes were treatment

---

[7]Walters JA, Tan DJ, White CJ, Gibson PG, Wood-Baker R. Systemic corticosteroids for acute exacerbations of chronic obstructive pulmonary disease. *Cochrane Database Syst Rev.* 2014;9:CD001288.

[8]Ceviker Y, Sayiner A. Comparison of two systemic steroid regimens for the treatment of COPD exacerbations. *Pulm Pharmacol Ther.* 2014;27(2):179-183.

[9]Walters JA, Tan DJ, White CJ, Wood-Baker R. Different durations of corticosteroid therapy for exacerbations of chronic obstructive pulmonary disease. *Cochrane Database Syst Rev.* 2018;3:CD006897.

failure (defined as the need for additional treatment or readmission through 2 weeks), relapse after treatment through 6 months, and adverse drug effects. There were no statistically significant differences in these outcomes or secondary outcomes (mortality, hospital length of stay) between shorter and longer duration groups. The generalizability of these results is limited by the absence of patients with mild or moderate COPD or mild exacerbations not requiring hospitalization.

These results were also largely influenced by the REDUCE trial,[10] a multicenter, double-blind, randomized controlled noninferiority trial of 314 patients randomized to short-term (5 days) versus conventional (14 days) corticosteroid therapy. REDUCE excluded asthma patients and included COPD patients with a >20 pack-year smoking history and ≥2 cardinal symptoms of COPD exacerbation. All patients received antibiotic therapy and were initially treated with 40 mg of IV methylprednisolone and transitioned to 40 mg of oral prednisone daily. At 6 months, primary (rate of and time to re-exacerbation) and secondary (all-cause mortality, need for mechanical ventilation) outcomes did not differ between short-term and conventional groups. Average hospital stay was shorter in the short-term group (8 vs. 9 days; $P = .04$). One criticism of REDUCE is that it employed a more stringent requirement for tobacco exposure than previous studies, resulting in a sicker patient population (90% GOLD stage 3 or 4) and limiting generalizability to patients with mild or moderate COPD. However, in clinical practice, extended steroid tapers are rarely considered in milder disease. Another limitation is that the REDUCE trial employed a more aggressive adjunctive treatment regimen (including a 7-day course of a broad-spectrum antibiotic; nebulized, short-acting bronchodilators 4-6 times daily; combined inhaled glucocorticoid and β-2 agonist; and tiotropium), resulting in a lower rate of treatment failure than expected based on previous trials. As a result, the study may have been underpowered to detect small differences in primary outcomes.

Collectively, results from these studies are reflected in guideline recommendations. The GOLD, NICE, and European Respiratory Society (ERS)/American Thoracic Society (ATS) guidelines all recommend oral over IV corticosteroids in patients with intact gastrointestinal

---

[10]Leuppi JD, et al. Short-term vs conventional glucocorticoid therapy in acute exacerbations of chronic obstructive pulmonary disease: the REDUCE Randomized Clinical Trial. *J Am Med Assoc*. 2013;309:2223-2231.

function,[4,5,11] and the GOLD guidelines recommend no longer than 5 to 7 days of steroids (level A, based on RCTs and a rich body of high-quality evidence without significant limitation or bias).

> You start the patient on prednisone 40 mg daily with a plan for a 5-day course. Several hours later, you are paged to the bedside by respiratory therapy. The patient is receiving a third nebulizer treatment but is persistently tachypneic with increased work of breathing. You are concerned about acute hypercapnic respiratory failure (AHRF) and obtain an arterial blood gas (ABG), which shows a pH of 7.32 and $PaCO_2$ of 55 mm Hg. You weigh options for respiratory support and consider noninvasive ventilation (NIV).

What is the role of NIV in patients with COPD exacerbations?

NIV should be the first-line mode of ventilation in patients who develop AHRF (arterial pH < 7.35, $PaCO_2$ > 45 mm Hg).

A recent meta-analysis[12] evaluated data from 17 RCTs with 1264 total patients hospitalized for AHRF from a COPD exacerbation. Studies were included if they had blood gas confirmation of AHRF (pH < 7.35, $PaCO_2$ > 45 mm Hg) and involved comparisons of bilevel NIV plus usual care versus usual care alone (which varied between studies but included interventions such as oxygen, bronchodilators, corticosteroids, antibiotics, diuretics, and heparin). Studies were excluded if they enrolled patients with prior NIV treatment or if the usual care group included any form of assisted ventilation. Primary outcome measures were mortality and need for endotracheal intubation. The authors further divided patients into predefined subgroups related to initial mean pH (<7.3 versus 7.3-7.35) and level of care (hospital ward versus ICU).

Compared to usual care, NIV decreased the risk of mortality (RR 0.54, 95% CI 0.38-0.76; P = .0005; NNT = 12) and intubation (RR 0.36, 95% CI 0.28-0.48; P < .00001; NNT = 5). Subgroup analysis

---

[11]Wedzicha JA, et al. Management of COPD exacerbations: a European Respiratory Society/American Thoracic Society guideline. *Eur Resp J.* 2017;49:1600791.

[12]Osadnik CR, et al. Non-invasive ventilation for the management of acute hypercapnic respiratory failure due to exacerbation of chronic obstructive pulmonary disease. *Cochrane Database Syst Rev.* 2017;(7):CD004104.

showed that these results were largely independent of initial pH or level of care. NIV was also associated with decreased length of hospital stay (mean difference −3.39 days, 95% CI −5.93 to −0.85; P = .009). A limitation of this meta-analysis is the lack of blinding in most trials, given the inherent difficulty of blinding with the treatment intervention.

The results from this meta-analysis are consistent with major society guidelines, which support use of NIV in patients with AHRF due to a COPD exacerbation. The GOLD guidelines[4] recommend NIV as the first-line mode of ventilation in patients with respiratory acidosis (arterial pH <7.35, $PaCO_2$ >45 mm Hg), severe dyspnea with clinical signs of respiratory muscle fatigue, or persistent hypoxemia despite supplemental oxygen therapy (level A, based on RCTs and a rich body of high-quality evidence without significant limitation or bias). The ERS/ATS guidelines[11] recommend use of NIV in all patients with AHRF (strong recommendation, low-quality evidence), and the NICE guidelines[5] recommend NIV as first line for persistent hypercapnic respiratory failure despite optimal medical treatment (grade A, based on evidence from systematic reviews or meta-analyses of RCTs).

You start the patient on bilevel NIV. His work of breathing and ABG subsequently improve. He is soon weaned off his ventilatory support and ultimately discharged on oral prednisone and levofloxacin.

KEY LEARNING POINTS

1. A sputum culture does not need to be routinely sent in patients with COPD exacerbations but should be considered in patients with severe underlying disease or those hospitalized for COPD exacerbations with purulent sputum or requiring ventilatory support.
2. Antibiotics should be given to all patients requiring ventilatory support as well as those with sputum purulence and at least one additional cardinal symptom of COPD exacerbation.
3. Oral corticosteroids administered for 5 days at a dose equivalent to 40 mg of prednisone are an appropriate therapeutic regimen for patients with COPD exacerbations.
4. NIV should be the first-line mode of ventilation in patients who develop AHRF (arterial pH < 7.35, $PaCO_2$ > 45 mm Hg).

VENOUS THROMBOEMBOLISM

Mehraneh Khalighi, MD

A 50-year-old woman with chronic obstructive pulmonary disease (COPD) presents with 1 week of left leg pain and swelling and new acute pleuritic chest pain associated with worsened shortness of breath. The ED provider obtains a CT pulmonary angiogram, which reveals the following:

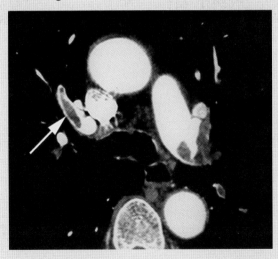

You diagnose the patient with acute pulmonary embolism (PE) and pursue left lower extremity venous doppler, which demonstrates an occlusive popliteal vein thrombosis. The patient's vital signs are stable, and she is not hypoxic.

She also denies history of malignancy, liver or kidney disease, bleeding, or thrombocytopenia. You are called to admit the patient to the hospital for treatment of her venous thromboembolism (VTE).

Can hospitalization be avoided in patients with acute symptomatic PE who are at low risk for complications?

In patients with low-risk PE and no bleeding risk factors such as severe liver or kidney disease, recent bleeding, or severe thrombocytopenia, treatment at home or early discharge is preferred over standard hospitalization.

The safety of outpatient treatment of patients with symptomatic PE at low risk for short-term adverse events or death was studied in a 2010 multicenter randomized clinical trial[1] of 132 patients with acute symptomatic PE. Low risk for complications from PE was defined as a risk score of ≤2 based on a previously proposed clinical prediction rule[2] (derived from clinical variables of recent major bleeding, metastatic cancer, Cr >2, cancer without metastasis, immobility, absence of surgery within 2 months, age >60 years). Patients were randomized to early discharge (on day 3 after right ventricular [RV] dysfunction was ruled out with transthoracic echocardiography [TTE] or day 5 if TTE could not be obtained) versus standard hospitalization (after the first 5 days of treatment) and followed for 3 months. Primary outcomes were nonfatal VTE recurrences, major and minor bleeding, and overall mortality.

The early discharge and standard hospitalization groups did not differ with respect to nonfatal VTE recurrence (2.8% vs. 3.3%, RR 0.83, 95% CI 0.12-5.74; P = .62), major (1.4% vs. 1.6%, RR 0.83, 95% CI 0.05-13.04; P = .70) and minor (4.2% vs. 3.3%, RR 1.25, 95% CI 0.22-7.24; P = .59) bleeding, or mortality (4.2% vs. 8.3%, RR 0.50, 95% CI 0.12-2.01; P = .26). However, the trial was suspended after a trend toward higher short-term mortality (within 10 days of diagnosis) was observed in the early discharge group. Study caveats include use of an unvalidated prognostic model for determining complication risk, which could have influenced observed differences in short-term mortality.

This question was subsequently evaluated in a 2011 open-label, multinational, randomized, noninferiority trial of 344 patients with

---

[1]Otero R, et al. Home treatment in pulmonary embolism. *Thromb Res.* 2010;126(1):e1-e5.
[2]Uresandi F, et al. A clinical prediction rule for identifying short-term risk of adverse events in patients with pulmonary thromboembolism. *Arch Bronconeumol.* 2007;43(11):617-622.

acute symptomatic PE and a low risk of death within 30 days.[3] The Pulmonary Embolism Severity Index (PESI) was utilized to define low risk (PESI class I or II). Patients presenting to EDs were randomized to outpatient versus inpatient PE treatment with subcutaneous enoxaparin followed by oral anticoagulation with a vitamin K antagonist. A noninferiority margin of 4% was used for defining a significant difference in outcomes between outpatient and inpatient treatment groups. The primary outcome was symptomatic, recurrent VTE within 90 days, and secondary outcomes included major bleeding within 14 and 90 days and 90-day all-cause mortality.

There was no difference in the primary outcome (0.6% with outpatient treatment vs. 0% with inpatient treatment, 95% upper confidence limit (UCL) for difference 2.7%; P = .011 for noninferiority). Outpatient treatment was also noninferior to inpatient treatment with respect to secondary outcomes.

A 2012 meta-analysis was conducted[4] to study the safety of outpatient treatment of patients with acute PE and at low risk for complications such as recurrent PE or bleeding. Studies were grouped into three categories: outpatient (13 studies representing 1657 patients in which patients were discharged within 24 hours), early discharge (3 studies representing 256 patients in which patients were discharged within 72 hours), and inpatient (5 studies representing 383 patients). Primary outcomes were 3-month recurrent VTE, major bleeding, and mortality. Although studies used different methods for defining low risk, most used comparable exclusion criteria for early discharge (e.g., high PESI index, large PE affecting >40% lung perfusion on V/Q scan or involving two or more lobar branches on imaging, hemodynamic and respiratory instability, evidence of RV strain based on TTE findings, or elevated troponin or N-terminal probrain natriuretic peptide [NT-proBNP] levels).

The pooled incidence of recurrent VTE in outpatient, early discharge, and inpatient categories were 1.70% (95% CI 0.92%-3.12%), 1.12% (95% CI 0.22%-5.43%), and 1.18% (95% CI 0.16%-8.14%), respectively (no P-values reported). The pooled incidence of major

---

[3]Aujesky D, et al. Outpatient versus inpatient treatment for patients with acute pulmonary embolism: an international, open-label, randomized, non-inferiority trial. *Lancet.* 2011;378(9785):41-48.

[4]Zondag W, et al. Outpatient versus inpatient treatment in patients with pulmonary embolism: a meta-analysis. *Eur Respir J.* 2013;42(1):134-144.

bleeding was 0.97% (95% CI 0.58%-1.59%) across outpatient studies, 0.78% (95% CI 0.16%-3.73%) across early discharge studies, and 1.04% (95% CI 0.39%-2.75%) across inpatient studies. Adjusting for underlying malignancy, the pooled incidence of mortality was 1.94% (95% CI 0.79%-4.84%) of patients in outpatient studies, 2.34% (95% CI 1.06%-5.12%) of patients in early discharge studies, and 0.74% (95% CI 0.04%-11.14%) of patients in inpatient studies.

Based on these collective results, the 2016 American College of Chest Physicians (ACCP) guidelines on antithrombotic therapy for VTE disease[5] suggest outpatient or early discharge treatment of clinically stable patients with good cardiopulmonary reserve over standard inpatient treatment in the absence of contraindications (e.g., recent bleeding, severe renal or liver disease, severe thrombocytopenia; class 2, level B). The use of clinical prediction rules such as the PESI is encouraged to identify low-risk patients.

> You determine that the patient is low risk using the PESI and discuss outpatient treatment. She lives alone and worries about going home without help. Via shared decision-making, you decide to observe her overnight in the hospital while she plans for family to stay with her after discharge. You notice that the ED provider has written several orders to expedite the admission, including an initial enoxaparin injection with plans to initiate warfarin later that evening.

Is warfarin still considered "standard therapy" for long-term anticoagulation for VTE in patients without cancer?

Nonvitamin K, direct-acting oral anticoagulants (DOACs) are preferred over vitamin K antagonists (VKAs) as long-term anticoagulant therapy in patients with VTE without cancer.

From 2012 to 2014, more than 20,000 patients were enrolled in several large randomized clinical trials—AMPLIFY, EINSTEIN-EF, Hokusai-VTE, and RECOVER II—that addressed this question by comparing the efficacy and safety of DOACs versus warfarin.

---

[5]Kearon C, et al. Antithrombotic therapy for VTE disease: CHEST guideline and expert panel report. *Chest.* 2016;149(2):315-352.

AMPLIFY[6] was a randomized double-blind noninferiority trial that compared efficacy and safety of apixaban to conventional therapy (subcutaneous enoxaparin followed by warfarin) in 5395 patients with acute VTE. The primary efficacy outcome of recurrent symptomatic VTE or VTE-related death occurred in 2.3% in the apixaban versus 2.7% in the conventional therapy group (RR 0.84, 95% CI 0.60-1.18; $P < .001$ for the prespecified noninferiority margin). The primary safety outcome of major bleeding was less frequent in the apixaban group (0.6% vs. 1.8%, RR 0.31, 95% CI 0.17-0.55; $P < .001$ for superiority). Similarly, the composite outcome of major bleeding or clinically relevant minor bleeding was less frequent in the apixaban group (4.3% vs. 9.7%, RR 0.44, 95% CI 0.36-0.55; $P < .001$ for superiority).

EINSTEIN-EF[7] was a randomized, open-label, noninferiority trial comparing rivaroxaban to conventional therapy (subcutaneous enoxaparin followed by warfarin) in 4832 patients with acute symptomatic PE with or without deep vein thrombosis (DVT). Rivaroxaban was noninferior to conventional therapy for the primary efficacy outcome of symptomatic recurrent VTE (2.1% vs. 1.8%, HR 1.12, 95% CI 0.75-1.68; $P = .003$ for noninferiority). The primary safety outcome of major or clinically relevant nonmajor bleeding was comparable across the groups (10.3% in the rivaroxaban group vs. 11.4% in the conventional therapy group, HR 0.90, 95% CI 0.76-1.07; $P = .23$). However, major bleeding occurred less frequently in the rivaroxaban group (1.1% vs. 2.2%, HR 0.49, 95% CI 0.31-0.79; $P = .003$).

Hokusai-VTE[8] investigators studied the noninferiority and safety of edoxaban versus conventional therapy (heparin followed by warfarin) in a randomized double-blind design. The trial enrolled 4921 patients with DVT and 3319 patients with PE (including 938 patients with PE associated with RV dysfunction as determined by NT-proBNP levels). Edoxaban was noninferior to conventional therapy with respect to the primary outcome of recurrent symptomatic VTE (3.2% vs. 3.5%,

[6]Agnelli G, et al. Oral apixaban for the treatment of acute venous thromboembolism. *N Engl J Med*. 2013;369(9):799-808.

[7]EINSTEIN-EF Investigators; Büller HR, et al. Oral rivaroxaban for the treatment of symptomatic pulmonary embolism. *N Engl J Med*. 2012;366(14):1287-1297.

[8]Hokusai-VTE Investigators; Büller HR, et al. Edoxaban versus warfarin for the treatment of symptomatic venous thromboembolism. *N Engl J Med*. 2013;369(15):1406-1415.

HR 0.89, 95% CI 0.70-1.13; $P < .001$ for noninferiority). However, the subset of patients with significant PE had a lower rate of recurrent VTE with edoxaban (3.3% vs. 6.2% in the conventional therapy group, HR 0.52, 95% CI 0.28-0.98; P-value not reported). The rate of major bleeding or clinically relevant nonmajor bleeding was lower in the edoxaban group (8.5% vs. 10.3%, HR 0.81, 95% CI 0.71-0.94; $P = .004$ for superiority).

Finally, in a randomized, double-blind, double-dummy trial, RECOVER II investigators[9] compared anticoagulation with dabigatran versus conventional therapy (low-molecular-weight or fractionated heparin followed by warfarin) for acute VTE in 2589 patients. Dabigatran was noninferior to warfarin with respect to the primary outcome: the composite of recurrent VTE or related death in 6 months (2.3% vs. 2.2%, HR 1.08, 95% CI 0.64-1.80; $P < .001$ for noninferiority). The groups did not differ in the safety outcome of major bleeding (1.2% in the dabigatran group vs. 1.7% in the conventional therapy group, HR 0.69, 95% CI 0.36-1.32; P-value not reported).

Collectively, these studies confirm that DOACs are noninferior to warfarin with respect to efficacy outcomes and safer with respect to bleeding outcomes. A common caveat is that time within therapeutic range (TTR) for warfarin therapy across these studies ranged between 59% and 64%, which is significantly higher than observed in real-world settings. The 2016 ACCP Chest guidelines on antithrombotic therapy for VTE disease[5] indicate that DOAC therapy is preferred over warfarin for initial treatment of patients with acute VTE who otherwise do not have contraindications to treatment with these agents (class 2, level B).

After discussion with the patient, you start her on rivaroxaban and she has an uneventful night. On morning rounds the next day, the patient complains of persistent left leg discomfort. Your medical student asks you if the patient should have an inferior vena cava (IVC) filter placed to prevent her from having more thromboembolic events.

[9]RECOVER II Investigators; Schulman S, et al. Treatment of acute venous thromboembolism with dabigatran or warfarin and pooled analysis. *Circulation*. 2014;129(7):764-772.

Does IVC filter placement reduce the risk of recurrent thromboembolism after an acute episode of VTE?

In addition to anticoagulation, IVC filter placement in patients with acute VTE does not reduce recurrent PE.

This question was studied by the PREPIC Study Group[10] in a randomized trial in which 400 patients with proximal DVT, with or without PE, were randomized to receive a permanent IVC filter in addition to standard anticoagulation versus standard anticoagulation alone for at least 3 months. Patients were followed for 8 years and outcome data for symptomatic PE, recurrent DVT, and postthrombotic syndrome (available for 99% of patients) were reviewed blindly by an independent committee.

Symptomatic PE was less frequent in the IVC filter group (6.2% vs. 15.1%, HR 0.37, 95% CI 0.17-0.79; P = .008), but recurrent DVT was more frequent (35.7% vs. 27.5%, HR 1.52, 95% CI 1.02-2.27; P = .042). Both postthrombotic syndrome (70.3% vs. 69.7%, HR 0.87, 98% CI 0.66-1.13; P = .30) and mortality at 8 years (48.1% vs. 51.0%, HR 0.97, 95% CI 0.50-1.42; P = .83) were comparable between the groups. Comparability to other studies and clinical extrapolation are limited by use of permanent IVC filters, which have fallen out of use.

In a subsequent study in 2015, the PREPIC2 Study Group[11] reported results from a randomized, open-label, blinded trial that evaluated 399 hospitalized patients with acute and symptomatic PE associated with lower extremity DVT and ≥1 severity criterion (defined as age >75 years, active cancer, chronic cardiac or respiratory insufficiency, ischemic stroke with leg paralysis within the last 6 months, DVT of the iliocaval segment or bilateral DVT, signs of RV dysfunction or myocardial injury). Patients were randomized to anticoagulation with or without a retrievable IVC filter. All patients were treated with full-dose anticoagulation for ≥6 months, and filter retrieval was planned at 3 months after placement. The primary outcome was recurrent fatal or

---

[10]The PREPIC Study Group. Eight-year follow-up of patients with permanent vena cava filters in the prevention of pulmonary embolism: the PREPIC (Prévention du Risque d'Embolie Pulmonaire par Interruption Cave) randomized study. *Circulation.* 2005;112:416-422.

[11]Mismetti P, et al. Effect of a retrievable inferior vena cava filter plus anticoagulation vs anticoagulation alone on risk of recurrent pulmonary embolism: a randomized clinical trial. *J Am Med Assoc.* 2015;313(16):1627-1635.

symptomatic nonfatal PE at 3 months, and secondary outcomes were recurrent fatal or symptomatic nonfatal PE at 6 months and new or recurrent symptomatic DVT at 3 and 6 months. Safety outcomes were major bleeding and death from any cause at 3 and 6 months and filter complications any time after insertion until retrieval.

Of 200 patients in the IVC filter group, 193 had successful filter implantation. Thirteen filter patients died within 3 months of insertion, and removal was not attempted in 15 patients because they were either too ill for the procedure, had filter thrombosis, or still needed the filter. One patient refused filter retrieval. Therefore, filter removal was attempted in 164 patients and successfully retrieved in 153 patients. There was no difference in the primary outcome (3% in the IVC filter group vs. 1.5% in the no filter group, RR 2.00; 95% CI 0.51-7.89; P = .50). Similarly, there was no difference in secondary outcomes. Filter complications included access site hematoma (2.6%), filter thrombosis (1.6%), and retrieval failure due to mechanical reasons (5.7%). One patient had cardiac arrest during filter insertion. Based on these studies, the 2016 ACCP Chest guidelines on antithrombotic therapy for VTE disease5 recommend against the use of IVC filter in patients with acute VTE or PE who are treated with anticoagulation (class 1, level B).

You explain to the patient and your medical student that IVC filter placement is not indicated because it does not decrease her risk of recurrent VTE and exposes her to possible procedural complications. The patient agrees with discharge to home after a brief observation stay.

KEY LEARNING POINTS

1. In patients with low-risk PE without risk factors for bleeding, treatment at home or early discharge is preferred over standard hospitalization.
2. Nonvitamin K, DOACs are preferred over VKAs as long-term anticoagulant therapy in patients with VTE without cancer.
3. In addition to anticoagulation, IVC filter placement in patients with acute VTE does not reduce recurrent PE.

INFECTIVE ENDOCARDITIS

Mara Bann, MD

You are called by the ED to evaluate a patient presenting with fever, tachycardia, and leukocytosis. The physician there has obtained a urinalysis and chest radiograph, neither of which reveals evidence of infection. The patient's past medical history is notable for intravenous drug use, and you note an apparently new cardiac murmur on physical examination. Suspecting infection as a source of the patient's signs and symptoms, the bedside nurse asks if you would like to draw blood cultures.

How do consecutive blood cultures obtained within a 24-hour period affect pathogen recovery?

Increasing the number of consecutive blood cultures up to as many as four sets of cultures over a 24-hour period increases pathogen recovery.

Widespread use of automated culturing systems over the last several decades necessitated the reevaluation of optimal blood culture sample collection protocols originally created in the late 1970s and 1980s. In a 2004 single-center retrospective study of 37,568 blood cultures obtained from adult patients tested on an automated culturing system, researchers evaluated the relationship between several testing parameters and pathogen recovery.[1] A blood culture was defined as blood obtained from one venipuncture divided equally and inoculated into a "set" of aerobic and anaerobic culture media bottles. Only positive cul-

---

[1]Cockerill FR, et al. Optimal testing parameters for blood cultures. *Clin Infect Dis.* 2004;38:1724-1730.

ture results thought to represent clinically relevant bloodstream infection were included. Culture positivity was defined based on the total number consecutive cultures drawn from the same patient in a 24-hour period. Given the association between infective endocarditis (IE) and degree of bacteremia, results were stratified by those with and without a clinical diagnosis of IE (based on medical chart review by treating physicians).

Of patients without clinical IE who had ≥3 cultures drawn, diagnostic yield increased with the number of consecutive cultures: 65% (106/163) of bloodstream infections were identified with the first culture, whereas 80.4% (131/163), 95.7% (156/163), and 100% (163/163) were identified with the second, third, and fourth cultures, respectively. Patients with clinical IE tended to have earlier blood culture positivity: 88.8% (16/18) had bloodstream infections identified with the first culture and 94.4% (17/18) with two cultures. Study caveats include single-center design and potential influence of local microbiologic patterns or clinical practice standards.

In 2007, a retrospective study replicated this analysis using similar sample collection, laboratory techniques, and study design in two geographically independent hospitals.[2] Only patients with ≥3 blood cultures drawn within a 24-hour period were included, and results were stratified by number of causative microorganisms identified (unimicrobial versus polymicrobial) but not clinical diagnosis of IE. This study corroborated previous findings, showing that diagnostic yield increases with the number of blood culture samples obtained. Of unimicrobial bloodstream infections for which ≥3 blood cultures were obtained, 73.1% (460/629) were identified with first culture, 89.7% (564/629) with two cultures, 98.2% (618/629) with three cultures, and 99.8% (628/629) with four cultures.

Neither study addressed timing of antimicrobial therapy in relation to culture acquisition, potentially confounding results, and detail about the timing of consecutive cultures within a 24-hour period was limited (e.g., frequently occurred within 30 minutes of each other in the first study; timing not reported in the second study). Nonetheless, based on the finding that higher numbers of consecutive blood cultures increase diagnostic yield, the 2015 American Heart Association (AHA)/Infectious Diseases Society of America (IDSA) endocarditis

---

[2]Lee A, et al. Detection of blood stream infections in adults: how many blood cultures are needed? *J Clin Microbiol.* 2007;45(11):3546-3548.

guidelines recommend that ≥3 sets of cultures be obtained from different venipuncture sites for patients with clinical suspicion of IE with the first and last samples drawn at least 1 hour apart (class I, level of evidence A).[3]

> Two sets of blood cultures are drawn in the ED, and you begin the patient on empiric antibiotic treatment for possible bacteremia and IE. You admit the patient to the hospital with the plan to repeat cultures within 24 hours. The next day, preliminary laboratory report results from blood cultures drawn in the ED identify gram-positive cocci. You obtain a transthoracic echocardiogram (TTE), which does not identify vegetation or other signs of IE. However, the study is deemed nondiagnostic due to poor image quality. You consider next steps for evaluating the source of the patient's presumed infection.

How definitive is the standard approach to interpreting TTE in ruling out IE?

TTE interpreted using a standard approach is inadequate for definitively ruling out IE.

This question was addressed in a 2016 single-center retrospective analysis[4] of 790 cases of suspected native-valve IE in which patients underwent both TTE and TEE within a 7-day period. Patients with high-risk clinical features such as prior valve repair or replacement, complex congenital disease, history of heart transplant, or indwelling devices were excluded. The authors compared two analysis approaches to TTE results: (1) a standard analysis involving presence or absence of vegetation versus (2) a set of strict negative rule-out criteria (moderate or better quality of ultrasound; normal valve anatomy; no valvular stenosis or sclerosis; at most trivial valvular regurgitation; at most mild, simple pericardial effusion; absence of implanted hardware or a central venous catheter; no vegetation). TEE was used as the gold-standard comparison.

---

[3]Baddour LM, et al. Infective endocarditis in adults: diagnosis, antimicrobial therapy, and management of complications: A scientific statement for healthcare professionals from the American Heart Association. *Circulation.* 2015;132(15):1435-1486.
[4]Sivak JA, et al. An approach to improve the negative predictive value and clinical utility of transthoracic echocardiography in suspected native valve infective endocarditis. *J Am Soc Echocardiogr.* 2016;29:315-322.

Using the standard approach, 661/790 TTE studies showed no evidence of vegetation compared to 104/790 negative TTE studies using the strict negative rule-out criteria. Compared to the strict negative rule-out criteria, the standard approach had lower sensitivity (43% [95% CI, 36%-51%] vs. 98% [95% CI, 95%-99%]; *P*-value not reported) and negative predictive value (87% [95% CI, 84%-89%] vs. 97% [95% CI, 92%-99%]; *P*-value not reported) for detection of vegetations. Therefore, despite its single-site scope and retrospective design, this study nonetheless demonstrated the inadequacy of standard TTE interpretation for definitively ruling out IE compared to TEE and underscored the need for additional evaluation. This concept aligns with 2015 ESC guidelines, [5] which recommend additional evaluation with TEE in all patients with clinical suspicion of IE and a negative or nondiagnostic TTE (class I, level of evidence B).

Based on the nondiagnostic TTE results, the patient undergoes TEE, which identifies a small aortic valve vegetation. There is mild aortic regurgitation but no perivalvular abscess or heart failure. You counsel the patient about the risk of systemic embolization, and he asks whether a medication like aspirin can prevent this.

What is the role of aspirin in preventing systemic embolic events among patients with IE?

Neither short- nor long-term aspirin use protects against embolic events in IE.

MATIE, a randomized, double-blinded, placebo-controlled trial, aimed to answer this question by randomizing 115 adult patients with IE from 19 centers to receive 4 weeks of aspirin (325 mg/d) versus placebo.[6] Patients between 16 and 80 years old were included if they met ≥2 of the following criteria: (1) ≥2 sets of positive blood cultures without known extracardiac source; (2) evidence of left-sided vegetation by echocardiogram; (3) ≥2 clinical findings consistent with endocarditis (fever, new or changing cardiac murmur, preexisting heart disease, microvascular findings). Both native-valve and prosthetic-valve endocarditis were included in the study. Exclusion criteria included isolated right-sided endocarditis, perivalvular abscess, probable surgical

---

[5]Habib G, et al. 2015 ESC guidelines for the management of infective endocarditis: the task force for the management of infective endocarditis of the European Society of Cardiology (ESC). *Eur Heart J*. 2015;36(44):3075-3128.
[6]Chan KL, et al. A randomized trial of aspirin on the risk of embolic events in patients with infective endocarditis. *J Am Coll Cardiol*. 2003;42(5):775-780.

intervention within the next 7 days, current aspirin use, recent stroke, or increased bleeding risk (e.g., active peptic ulcer disease within the past 12 months, history of bleeding diathesis).

The primary outcome—clinical embolism to the brain or other organs—was assessed by regular history and physical examination during hospitalization and at outpatient follow-up. New neurologic deficits were evaluated and categorized as embolic versus hemorrhagic via neurologist assessment and CT of the brain. All patients received TTE at baseline and completion of antibiotic therapy. Secondary outcomes included death, subclinical stroke, major or minor bleeding, valvular surgery, and vegetation progression (number/size of vegetation or severity of valvular dysfunction by TTE).

There was no difference in the primary outcome between high-dose aspirin and placebo groups (28.3% vs. 20.0%, respectively, OR 1.62, 95% CI, 0.68-3.86; $P = .29$). Similarly, secondary outcomes did not vary by treatment group. Post-hoc analysis[7] comparing 84 patients excluded because of long-term daily aspirin to 55 patients randomized to placebo demonstrated no statistically significant impact of long-term aspirin therapy on risk of embolism (OR 0.91, 95% CI, 0.40-2.07; $P = .825$). Study limitations include underenrollment and issues with study power.

In coordination with an infectious disease consultant, you recommend a long-term intravenous antibiotic treatment course targeted to culture and sensitivity results. You plan for him to remain hospitalized for several weeks to complete therapy. You develop a substance use disorder management plan with the patient and an addiction medicine specialist.

You rotate off-service and when you return 2 weeks later, he confides that he feels more fatigued than when you first admitted him to the hospital. He does not have symptoms at rest but notes significant shortness of breath with regular physical activity. You are surprised at how dyspneic he becomes with ambulation to the nurses' station. Repeat TTE shows severe aortic regurgitation with dilation of the left ventricle and moderately depressed ejection fraction. You express concern that he may need valvular surgery and suggest discussing this plan with a cardiac surgeon. He is very worried and tells you that he does not wish to undergo surgery unless absolutely necessary.

---

[7]Chan KL, et al. Effect of long-term aspirin use on embolic events in infective endocarditis. *Clin Infect Dis.* 2008;46(1):37-41.

What is the benefit of valvular surgery for patients with IE and heart failure?

Valvular surgery is associated with a survival benefit in patients with left-sided IE complicated by heart failure, with the greatest benefit among those with moderate to severe heart failure (New York Heart Association [*NYHA*] *class III or IV symptoms*).

A 2003 retrospective observational cohort study evaluated 513 cases of complicated left-sided native-valve endocarditis at seven hospitals.[8] Patients were qualified for the study by meeting Duke criteria for definite or possible endocarditis and experiencing a clinical complication for which valve surgery would be considered (heart failure, new valvular regurgitation, refractory infection, systemic embolization, or presence of vegetation on echocardiography). Propensity score matching (between patients undergoing valve surgery versus receiving medical therapy) was also used to address selection bias. Exclusion criteria included comatose state and absence of follow-up outcome data. In total, 45% (230/513) of patients underwent at least one valve surgery, including mechanical valve replacement (109/230, 47%), bioprosthetic-valve replacement (102/230, 44%), or valve repair (20/230, 9%). The primary outcome was 6-month mortality.

After multivariable adjustment, valve surgery was associated with decreased mortality (HR 0.35, 95% CI, 0.23-0.54; $P < .05$). Propensity score-matched analysis of 218 patients (109 undergoing valve surgery, 109 unique control patients) showed an association between valve surgery and decreased mortality (15% vs. 28% in control group, HR 0.45, 95% CI 0.23-0.86; $P < .05$). Propensity-matched subgroup analysis demonstrated that mortality reduction with surgery versus medical therapy was most pronounced in patients with moderate to severe heart failure (14% vs. 51% with less severe heart failure, HR 0.22, 95% CI 0.09-0.53; $P < .05$).

In 2011, researchers used data from the International Collaboration on Endocarditis Prospective Cohort Study (ICE-PCS)—which enrolled patients with IE from 61 centers across 28 countries—to further investigate the association between valvular surgery and mortality for patients with IE and heart failure. In this prospective cohort study of 4075 patients with definite IE by Duke criteria,[9] 1359 had heart failure (stratified by NYHA class), and 839 (61.7%) of the patients with heart failure

---

[8]Vikram HR, et al. Impact of valve surgery on 6-month mortality in adults with complicated, left-sided native valve endocarditis: a propensity analysis. *J Am Med Assoc.* 2003;290(24):3207-3214.
[9]Kiefer T, et al. Association between valvular surgery and mortality among patients with infective endocarditis complicated by heart failure. *J Am Med Assoc.* 2011;306(20):2239-2247.

underwent valvular surgery. In comparison, 1168 (43%) of the 2716 patients without heart failure underwent valvular surgery. The primary outcomes were mortality during hospitalization and at 1 year.

Compared to those receiving medical management, patients receiving surgery had lower in-hospital (OR 0.66, 95% CI 0.56-0.77; *P*-value not reported) and 1-year mortality (RR 0.50, 95% CI, 0.43-0.57; *P* < .001). Caveats include clinical diagnosis of heart failure and lack of information about timing of heart failure symptom onset or association between timing of surgery and study outcomes. Nonetheless, these findings are consistent with 2016 AATS guidelines [10] that recommend surgery during initial hospitalization for patients with IE who present with valve dysfunction resulting in heart failure symptoms (class 1, level of evidence B). These guidelines also recommend that decision-making about surgery and overall patient management account for addiction and include addiction treatment (class IIa, level of evidence C).

> You refer your patient to a cardiac surgeon. He undergoes valvular surgery with no complications. After completing a full course of intravenous antibiotics and physical therapy, he regains his functional tolerance and resumes his previous activity level.

KEY LEARNING POINTS

1. Increasing the number of consecutive blood cultures up to as many as four sets of cultures over a 24-hour period increases pathogen recovery.
2. TTE interpreted using a standard approach is inadequate for definitively ruling out IE.
3. Neither short- nor long-term aspirin use protects against embolic events in IE.
4. Valvular surgery is associated with a survival benefit in patients with left-sided IE complicated by heart failure, with the greatest benefit among those with moderate to severe heart failure (NYHA class III or IV symptoms).

---

[10]Pettersson GB, et al. 2016 The American Association for Thoracic Surgery (AATS) consensus guidelines: Surgical treatment of infective endocarditis: executive summary. *J Thorac Cardiovasc Surg.* 2017;153(6):1241-1258.

DELIRIUM

Erin Wu, MD,
Maya Narayanan, MD, MPH

You admit an ill-appearing 80-year-old man directly from clinic for community-acquired pneumonia. His breathing improves with 3 liters of supplemental oxygen, and you start intravenous antibiotics. Given his presenting illness and long list of home medications, you are mindful of his delirium risk.

What is the most effective strategy to prevent acute delirium in the hospital?

A multicomponent nonpharmacologic intervention that promotes mobility, maintains day-night cycle, optimizes nutrition and hydration, and improves vision/hearing impairment is the most effective method to prevent delirium.

This question was addressed in a prospective cohort study comparing 852 hospitalized elderly patients (age ≥70 years) who either received usual care or interventions related to six major delirium risk factors (Table 20.1).[1] Patients were matched according to age, sex, and baseline delirium risk (using a predictive model that defined high risk of delirium as 3-4 and intermediate risk as 1-2 of the following risk factors: visual impairment, severe illness, cognitive impairment, and high BUN:Cr ratio).

In the study group, a trained interdisciplinary team carried out the interventions (Table 20.1). All patients were evaluated daily for delirium using the digit span test, Mini-Mental State Examination (MMSE),

---

[1] Inouye SK, et al. A multicomponent intervention to prevent delirium in hospitalized older patients. *N Engl J Med.* 1999;340(9):669-676.

TABLE 20.1

Delirium Risk Factors and Corresponding Interventions

Delirium Risk Factor	Interventions
Cognitive impairment: MMSE score <20	Orientation with board listing names of care team members and day's schedule; reorient to surroundings; cognitively stimulating activities (word games)
Sleep deprivation	Sleep protocol including offering warm milk or herbal tea, relaxing music, back massage; hospital unit noise reduction
Immobility	Ambulation or active range of motion exercises three times daily; minimizing immobilizing equipment (catheters, restraints)
Visual impairment (<20/70 visual acuity)	Glasses or magnifying lenses, large print books, fluorescent tape on call bell
Hearing impairment (≤6 of 12 on whisper test)	Portable amplifying devices, earwax disimpaction
Dehydration: BUN:Cr ratio ≥ 18	Encouragement of oral fluid intake

MMSE, Mini-Mental State Examination.

and Confusion Assessment Method (CAM). The primary outcome was delirium defined by CAM criteria. Secondary outcomes included the total number of days with delirium, delirium recurrence (≥2 episodes), and delirium severity (defined by the number of delirium characteristics present: symptoms fluctuation, inattention, disorganized thinking, and altered level of consciousness).

Delirium was less common in the study group (10% vs. 15%; OR 0.60, 95% CI 0.39-0.92; P = .02), as was the total number of days of delirium (105 vs. 161 days; P = .02). Groups did not differ with respect to delirium recurrence or severity.

These findings are supported by a 2015 meta-analysis that evaluated 4267 patients from across 11 studies (4 randomized controlled trials and 7 nonrandomized studies, most of which used nonmatched or historical controls).[2] All studies implemented nonpharmacologic

---

[2]Hshieh TT, et al. Effectiveness of multicomponent nonpharmacologic delirium interventions: a meta-analysis. *J Am Med Assoc.* 2015;175(4):512-520.

interventions addressing one or more of the following factors: cognition or orientation, mobility, hearing, sleep-wake cycle, vision, and/or hydration and examined the effect on delirium incidence. The meta-analysis showed that the odds of delirium was lower in the intervention group compared to controls (OR 0.47, 95% CI 0.38-0.58; $P < .001$).

Collectively, these results align with the 2010 National Institute for Health and Clinical Excellence (NICE) guidelines on delirium prevention, which recommend "assessment and modification of key clinical factors that may precipitate delirium, including cognitive impairment or disorientation, dehydration or constipation, hypoxia, infection, immobility or limited mobility, several medications, pain, poor nutrition, sensory impairment, and sleep disturbance."[3]

You initiate a multicomponent nonpharmaceutical intervention that includes intravenous fluids, increasing daytime activity, and frequent reorientation. However, you receive a page overnight stating that your patient appears increasingly confused. His nurse is concerned that he is not responding to her questions appropriately and overhears him speaking out loud to an empty room. You assess the patient, who has a nonfocal neurological examination and no evidence of a fall. He is breathing comfortably, saturating well on 2 to 3 liters of supplemental oxygen. Laboratory testing does not reveal toxic-metabolic etiologies that could explain his confusion. You suspect acute delirium.

What instruments may be used to diagnose acute delirium in the hospital?

Among instruments, the CAM possesses the best evidence for diagnosing acute delirium in the inpatient setting.

The CAM was developed through a consensus building process by an expert panel and involves four "cardinal elements" (Table 20.2), with the diagnosis of delirium requiring the presence of features 1 and 2 as well as either 3 or 4. The CAM was prospectively validated through

---

[3]National Institute for Health and Clinical Excellence. *Delirium: diagnosis, prevention and management (NICE guideline 103)*; 2010. Available at: https://www.nice.org.uk/guidance/cg103/resources/delirium-prevention-diagnosis-and-management-pdf-35109327290821. Accessed September 30, 2018.

TABLE 20.2

Elements of the CAM and Corresponding Questions

Elements	Questions
1. Acute onset and fluctuating course	This element is usually obtained from a family member or nurse and is shown by positive responses to the following questions: • Is there evidence of an acute change in mental status from the patient's baseline? • Did the (abnormal) behavior fluctuate during the day, that is, tend to come and go, or increase and decrease in severity?
2. Inattention	This element is shown by a positive response to the following question: • Did the patient have difficulty focusing attention, for example, being easily distractible or having difficulty keeping track of what was being said?
3. Disorganized thinking	This element is shown by a positive response to the following question: • Was the patient's thinking disorganized or incoherent, such as rambling or irrelevant conversation, unclear or illogical flow of ideas, or unpredictable switching from subject to subject?
4. Altered level of consciousness	This element is shown by any answer other than "alert" to the following question: • Overall, how would you rate this patient's level of consciousness? Alert (normal), vigilant (hyperalert), lethargic (drowsy, easily aroused), stupor (difficult to arouse), or coma (unarousable).

a study conducted at two American academic medical centers[4] that involved CAM testing for a total of 26 patients with delirium (based on psychiatrist diagnosis) and 30 without. There was high interobserver reliability for CAM scoring (kappa = 0.81-1.0). Across study sites (site 1/site 2), the CAM was found to have a sensitivity of 94/100%, specificity of 90/95%, positive predictive value of 91/94%, and negative predictive value of 90/100%.

---

[4]Inouye SK, et al. Clarifying confusion. *Ann Intern Med.* 1990;113(12):941-948.

These findings were supported by a subsequent 2013 systematic review and meta-analysis evaluating the CAM and the CAM-ICU (a variation of the CAM developed for the critical care setting) among 1033 patients across nine studies,[5] which demonstrated a pooled sensitivity of 82% and specificity of 99%. Though the diagnosis of delirium must be made in conjunction with the clinical assessment, these results inform the 2010 NICE guidelines[6] supporting CAM as one of the best available instruments.

You diagnose your patient with delirium, which you suspect is multifactorial due to pneumonia, hypovolemia, and hospital-based factors (e.g., nighttime interruptions). In spite of antibiotics and continued nonpharmaceutical interventions, you receive a page that afternoon stating that he is trying to get out of bed and pull on his IV lines. His nurse inquires about the utility of pharmacologic therapy.

What are the roles of first- and second-generation antipsychotics (FGAs and SGAs) in the treatment of acute inpatient delirium?

FGAs and SGAs can be useful in treating acute inpatient delirium after conservative and preventative measures fail. SGAs may have slightly more favorable side-effect profiles.

A 2016 meta-analysis[7] addressed this question by incorporating data from 949 patients across 15 randomized controlled trials. Most studies were high-quality using the Cochrane risk-of-bias criteria. Patients were categorized as either receiving antipsychotics, usual care, or placebo. Four categorical meta-analyses were performed (pooled antipsychotics

---

[5]Shi Q, et al. Confusion assessment method: a systematic review and meta-analysis of diagnostic accuracy. *Neuropsychiatr Dis Treat.* 2013;9:1359-1370.

[6]National Institute for Healthcare and Excellence. Delirium: prevention, diagnosis, management. *Clinical Guideline [CG 103].* July 2010. Available at: https://www.nice.org.uk/guidance/cg103. Accessed September 14, 2019.

[7]Kishi T, et al. Antipsychotic medications for the treatment of delirium: a systematic review and meta-analysis of randomised controlled trials. *J Neurol Neurosurg Psychiatry.* 2016;87:767-774.

versus placebo/usual care, haloperidol versus SGAs, head-to-head comparisons of SGAs, and a single study comparing haloperidol to chlorpromazine). The primary outcome for each of the above comparisons was the delirium response rate, which was individually defined by the original studies based on severity of delirium scales or global scales. Secondary outcomes included delirium severity, scores on the Clinical Global Impression-Severity Scale (CGI-S), mortality, adverse effects, and time to response.

Treatment with antipsychotics led to superior response rates compared to placebo or usual care groups (RR = 0.22, 95% CI 0.15-0.34; $P < .001$). Antipsychotic therapy was also associated with reduced delirium severity scores ($P = .03$), CGI-S scores ($P < .001$), and time-to-response rates ($P < .001$). Antipsychotic therapy was also associated with increased frequency of side effects such as dry mouth and sedation ($P = .01$). Secondary pooled analysis demonstrated that extrapyramidal symptoms were more frequent and lasted longer with haloperidol versus SGAs ($P = .02$). Study caveats include inclusion of unpublished conference abstracts and studies conducted in ICU settings, author disclosures regarding pharmaceutical company compensation, need for caution among patients with or without risk factors for QTc prolongation (which was not addressed in the study).

Nonetheless, by providing evidence about short-term antipsychotic use for acute delirium, this meta-analysis has been built on evidence of a negative association between long-term antipsychotic use for dementia-related psychosis and mortality risk.[8-11] This study also balances findings from another meta-analysis that did not demonstrate a morbidity benefit but had limitations (e.g., high heterogeneity of included studies, inclusion of studies investigating prophylactic treatment of delirium[12]).

---

[8]Seitz D, et al. Antipsychotics in the treatment of delirium: A systematic review. *J Clin Psychiatry.* 2007;68(1):11-21.

[9]Lonergan E, et al. Antipsychotics for delirium. *Cochrane Database Syst Rev.* 2007(2):CD005594.

[10]Schneeweiss S, et al. Risk of death associated with the use of conventional versus atypical antipsychotic drugs among elderly patients. *Can Med Assoc J.* 2007;176(5):627-632.

[11]Schneider LS, et al. Risk of death with atypical antipsychotic drug treatment for dementia. meta-analysis of randomized placebo-controlled trials. *J Am Med Assoc.* 2005;294(15):1934-1943.

[12]Neufeld KJ, et al. Antipsychotic medication for prevention and treatment of delirium in hospitalized adults: a systematic review and meta-analysis. *J Am Geriatr Soc.* 2016;64:705-714.

While more investigation and data are needed, there can be benefit to antipsychotics as treatment for acute, agitated delirium after nonpharmacologic measures fail.

That night, you order quetiapine 25 mg orally, which helps with the patient's agitation and sleep. Over a few days, his mental status improves and quetiapine is discontinued. Due to his deconditioning from his pneumonia and acute delirium, he is discharged to a skilled nursing facility.

Are there long-term sequelae after acute delirium in the hospital?

Patients who suffer acute inpatient delirium are at increased risk of continued antipsychotic use, institutionalization, dementia, and death well after hospital discharge.

Two prospective observational studies evaluated the long-term (up to 1 year post discharge) outcomes of patients who experienced acute delirium in the hospital. One study conducted at a single Canadian hospital screened patients age ≥65 years who were admitted to the medical service for delirium; 243 patients were diagnosed with delirium at enrollment or within 1 week of admission and were compared to 118 other patients on the medical service who never had delirium.[13] One-year mortality was higher among patients in the delirium cohort (41.6% vs. 14.4%; $P < .001$). In multivariable analysis adjusted for age, sex, marital status, comorbidity, clinical severity of illness, and physical function, delirium was also associated with a twofold increase in mortality compared to controls (HR 2.11, 95% CI 1.18-3.77; $P < .05$). The risk of mortality for patients who experienced acute hospital delirium was examined at different intervals from discharge (month 1, months 2-6, and months 7-12 after discharge), and analysis showed equal risk of mortality for all time periods ($P = .70$).

The other study, conducted at a US academic medical center, enrolled patients age ≥70 years who were admitted to the general medicine service, did not have delirium on admission, and were at

---

[13]McCusker J, et al. Delirium predicts 12-month mortality. *Arch Intern Med.* 2002;162:457-463.

intermediate or high risk for delirium. The patients were followed for 1 year post discharge to evaluate the impact of acute inpatient delirium on rates of institutionalization or death.[14] Of the 433 patients enrolled, 378 never had delirium during their hospital stay and were compared to 31 patients with delirium that resolved by the time of hospital discharge and 24 patients with delirium at discharge. Delirium was defined using CAM criteria.

Patients with delirium at discharge had the highest rate of nursing home placement or death, followed by patients whose delirium had resolved at the time of discharge and patients without delirium (83.3% vs. 67.7% vs. 41.5%, $P < .001$). After adjusting for age, marital status, dementia, depression, activities of daily living impairment, and Charlson Comorbidity Index, the risk of institutionalization or death was higher for patients with delirium at discharge (HR 2.64, 95% CI 1.60-4.35; $P < .001$) and those whose delirium had resolved by time of discharge (HR 1.53, 95% CI 0.96-2.43; $P < .001$) compared with patients who did not have acute delirium.

These results were corroborated by a 2010 meta-analysis[15] evaluating the impact of acute delirium in the hospital on mortality, institutionalization, or dementia on 2957 patients across 42 studies that included one of these three outcomes of interest. Patients who experienced acute delirium in the hospital had a greater risk of death (HR 1.95, 95% CI 1.51-2.52; $P < .001$), institutionalization (OR 2.41, 95% CI 1.77-3.29; $P < .001$), and incident dementia (OR 12.52, 95% CI 1.86-84.21, $P = .009$) than patients who did not experience acute delirium). The data about acute delirium and poor long-term outcomes emphasize the importance of close primary care follow-up.

Several weeks later, the patient is discharged home from the skilled nursing facility. He continues to have mild cognitive impairment, but his respiratory status is back to baseline. His family makes an appointment for him to see his primary care physician in a few days.

---

[14]McAvay GJ, et al. Older adults discharged from the hospital with delirium: 1 year outcomes. *J Am Geriatr Soc.* 2006;54(8):1245-1250.

[15]Witlox J, et al. Delirium in elderly patients and the risk of postdischarge mortality, institutionalization and dementia: a meta-analysis. *J Am Med Assoc.* 2010;304(4):443-451.

KEY LEARNING POINTS

1. A multicomponent nonpharmacologic intervention that promotes mobility, maintains day-night cycle, optimizes nutrition and hydration, and improves vision/hearing impairment is the most effective method to prevent delirium.
2. Among instruments, the CAM possesses the best evidence for diagnosing acute delirium in the inpatient setting.
3. FGAs and SGAs can be useful in treating acute inpatient delirium after conservative and preventative measures fail. SGAs may have slightly more favorable side-effect profiles.
4. Patients who suffer acute inpatient delirium are at increased risk of continued antipsychotic use, institutionalization, dementia, and death well after hospital discharge.

END-STAGE LIVER DISEASE

Elijah J. Mun, MD,
Tyler J. Albert, MD

You are called by the ED to admit a 55-year-old man with history of cirrhosis secondary to chronic alcoholism complicated by hepatic encephalopathy (HE) and ascites who is brought in by his caregiver with increasing confusion, lethargy, and abdominal pain over 5 days. His caregiver reports the patient has completely abstained from alcohol for the past 4 months and is adherent to lactulose with daily bowel movements.

You perform a bedside ultrasound exam in the ED, which demonstrates the following (Figure 21.1).

You perform abdominal paracentesis and diagnose the patient with spontaneous bacterial peritonitis (SBP). Other laboratory and radiographic evaluations do not reveal any other potential causes of his symptoms. You initiate empiric IV antibiotics while awaiting ascitic fluid culture results and consider the role of albumin infusion.

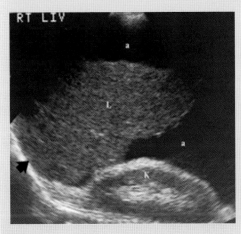

Figure 21.1 Cirrhosis and ascites. The liver (L) appears to be shrunken, nodular, and surrounded by ascites (a). The bare area of the liver (arrow) is closely applied to the diaphragm. The right kidney (K) is also seen in this image. (Reprinted from Brant W. *The Core Curriculum: Ultrasound.* Philadelphia: Lippincott Williams & Wilkins; 2001, with permission.)

What is the role of albumin infusion in the treatment of SBP?

In cirrhotic patients with SBP and Cr > 1 mg/dL, BUN > 30 mg/dL, or total bilirubin > 4 mg/dL, albumin infusion is associated with lower risk of renal failure and death.

This question was studied in a multicenter randomized controlled trial of 126 adult patients[1] diagnosed with SBP (based on ascitic fluid Polymorphonuclear cell count >250 cells/mm^3 in the absence of findings concerning for secondary bacterial peritonitis). Patients were randomized to receive either antibiotics alone (cefotaxime) or antibiotics (cefotaxime) plus IV albumin. Antibiotics were dosed based on patients' serum Cr and albumin was given twice—at the time of diagnosis (1.5 g/kg) and again 48 hours later on day 3 (1 g/kg). Exclusion criteria included antibiotic exposure within 1 week of SBP diagnosis, other infection, shock, gastrointestinal bleeding, ileus, grade 3 to 4 HE, or cardiac failure. Primary outcomes were renal impairment (defined as nonreversible deterioration of renal function during hospitalization) and mortality (in-hospital and 3-month).

Renal impairment was lower among patients in the antibiotics plus albumin group (10% vs. 33%; $P = .002$). Patients receiving antibiotics and albumin also had lower in-hospital (10% vs. 29%; $P = .01$) and 3-month (22% vs. 41%; $P = .03$) mortality. Baseline total bilirubin and Cr levels independently predicted renal impairment and in-hospital mortality, and among patients with total bilirubin <4 g/dL and Cr < 1 g/dL, renal impairment was less frequent in the antibiotics plus albumin group (0% vs. 7%; P-value not reported). Caveats include absent data about adequateness of fluid resuscitation or vasoconstrictor therapy among control group patients.

Other work has built upon these findings by demonstrating the acceptability of therapeutic protocols that utilize a restrictive strategy of administering albumin only to patients with high risk of renal failure (Cr>1, BUN >30, or total bilirubin >4)[2]—the strategy recommended in the 2014 AASLD practice guidelines (Class IIa, Level B recommendation).[3]

[1]Sort P, et al. Effect of intravenous albumin on renal impairment and mortality in patients with cirrhosis and spontaneous bacterial peritonitis. *N Engl J Med.* 1999;341(6):403-409.
[2]Sigal SH, et al. Restricted use of albumin for spontaneous bacterial peritonitis. *Gut.* 2007;56(4):597-599.
[3]Runyon BA. Introduction to the revised American Association for the Study of Liver Diseases Practice Guideline management of adult patients with ascites due to cirrhosis 2012. *Hepatology.* 2013;57(4):1651-1653.

Based on a serum Cr of 2.0 mg/dL, you treat the patient with IV albumin in addition to antibiotics. The patient gradually improves over the next few days, and you are asked by his caregiver if anything can be done to prevent such infections in the future.

In which situations should prophylactic antibiotics be considered for the prevention of SBP?

Prophylactic antibiotics should be initiated in cirrhotic patients with either gastrointestinal bleeding, previous SBP, or ascites if ascitic fluid protein <1 g/dL or ascitic fluid protein <1.5 g/dL and Child class C disease.

A meta-analysis evaluated five randomized controlled trials investigating the role of prophylactic antibiotics in cirrhotic patients with gastrointestinal bleeding.[4] Trials without control groups or those comparing two or more antibiotics were excluded. Four main efficacy outcomes were identified: proportion of patients free of infection, bacteremia and/or SBP, SBP, and death. The five trials accounted for a total of 534 patients, 264 of whom were treated with antibiotics for 4 to 10 days and 270 who did not receive antibiotics. Antibiotic prophylaxis was associated with a greater proportion of patients free of infection (32% mean rate difference, 95% CI 22%-42%; $P < .001$), bacteremia and/or SBP (19% mean rate difference, 95% CI 11%-26%; $P < .001$), SBP (7% mean rate difference, 95% CI 2.1%-12.6%; $P = .006$), and death (9.1% mean rate difference, 95% CI 2.9%-15.3%; $P = .004$).

Subsequent trials have also shown prophylactic antibiotics to be effective in the prevention of SBP in cirrhotic patients with previous SBP (SBP recurrence rate 35% among controls vs. 12% in those treated with norfloxacin; $P = .014$)[5] and ascites with ascitic fluid protein <1 g/dL or ascitic fluid protein <1.5 g/dL and Child-Pugh score >9, i.e., Child class C disease (comparing those treated with norfloxacin vs. controls, 1-year incidence of SBP 7% vs. 61%, $P < .001$; hepatorenal syndrome [HRS] 28% vs. 41%, $P = .02$; 3-month survival 94% vs. 62%, $P = .003$).[6]

---

[4]Bernard B, et al. Antibiotic prophylaxis for the prevention of bacterial infections in cirrhotic patients with gastrointestinal bleeding: a meta-analysis. *Hepatology.* 1999;29(6):1655-1661.
[5]Ginés P, et al. Norfloxacin prevents spontaneous bacterial peritonitis recurrence in cirrhosis: Results of a double-blind, placebo-controlled trial. *Hepatology.* 1990;12(4):716-724.
[6]Fernández J, et al. Primary prophylaxis of spontaneous bacterial peritonitis delays hepatorenal syndrome and improves survival in cirrhosis. *Gastroenterology.* 2007;133(3):818-824.

Consequently, AASLD guidelines recommend the administration of prophylactic antibiotics for any cirrhotic patients with gastrointestinal bleeding, previous SBP, and ascites if ascitic fluid protein <1 g/dL, or ascitic fluid protein <1.5 g/dL and Child class C disease (Class I, Level A).[3]

The patient and his caregiver agree to initiate daily oral norfloxacin for SBP prevention after hospital discharge. However, the patient continues to demonstrate mild lethargy and disorientation to time and place. You observe asterixis on physical examination and weigh whether to further titrate his lactulose or initiate rifaximin for treating his HE.

What is the role of rifaximin versus lactulose in the treatment of overt HE?

Rifaximin does not appear to be superior to lactulose, which remains the first-line option for treating HE.

Rifaximin and lactulose were compared in a meta-analysis that included five randomized controlled trials representing a total of 264 patients with an episode of overt HE, 136 of whom received rifaximin and 128 of whom received lactulose/lactitol.[7] Inclusion criteria included full length peer-reviewed articles evaluating patients aged ≥18 years, with serum ammonia levels ≥75 μmol/L, signs and symptoms of acute, chronic, or minimal HE according to Conn's modification of Parsons Smith classification.[8] Exclusion criteria included noncontrolled clinical trials, major psychiatric illness, chronic renal/respiratory insufficiency, tumors, concurrent infections, known hypersensitivity to rifaximin and/or nonabsorbable disaccharides, or treatment with sedatives or antibiotics within 7 days of study start date.

The primary outcome was clinical efficacy, which was defined as either improvement to a lower stage of HE or significant difference in portosystemic encephalopathy index (a measure that combines assessment of mental status and asterixis, along with electroencephalography,

---

[7]Jiang Q, et al. Rifaximin versus nonabsorbable disaccharides in the management of hepatic encephalopathy: a meta-analysis. *Eur J Gastroenterol Hepatol.* 2008;20(11):1064-1070.
[8]Conn HO, et al. Comparison of lactulose and neomycin in the treatment of chronic portal-systemic encephalopathy: a double blind controlled trial. *Gastroenterology.* 1977;72(4):573-583.

number connection test, and arterial ammonia level). Secondary outcomes included adverse events. The rifaximin and lactulose/lactitol groups did not vary with respect to clinical efficacy (pooled RR 1.08, 95% CI 0.85-1.38; $P = .53$). No serious adverse events were reported. Study caveats included heterogeneity in acuity, grade, or stage of HE and duration of therapy across studies.

AASLD guidelines recommend lactulose as the first choice for treatment of overt HE (Class I, Level B).[9] Rifaximin may be used as adjunctive therapy or when patients are unable to tolerate lactulose.

> You uptitrate the patient's lactulose to a goal of three to five bowel movements daily. He responds well and exhibits significant clinical improvement in HE signs and symptoms. Unfortunately, over the next several days, his urine output decreases and his serum Cr rises dramatically. His Cr fails to improve despite diuretic withdrawal and albumin challenge. After additional workup and input from the nephrology consult service, you diagnose him with HRS. You weigh initiating a vasoconstrictor.

What is the role of vasoconstrictors in the management of HRS?

Numerous vasoconstrictors have been shown to be beneficial in increasing mean arterial pressure (MAP) among patients with HRS. There is no convincing evidence of one vasoconstrictor being superior to another.

This question was addressed in a pooled analysis of 501 patients across 21 randomized and nonrandomized studies to evaluate whether treatment with a vasoconstrictor in HRS was associated with a rise in arterial blood pressure and recovery of kidney function.[10] Studies evaluated multiple vasoconstrictors, including terlipressin (used in most studies included in the pooled analysis), norepinephrine, octreotide, midodrine, ornipressin, and dopamine. Inclusion criteria included diagnosis of HRS

---

[9]Vilstrup H, et al. Hepatic encephalopathy in chronic liver disease: 2014 practice guideline by the American Association for the Study of Liver Diseases and the European Association for the Study of the Liver. *Hepatology.* 2014;60(2):715-735.

[10]Velez JCQ, Nietert PJ. Therapeutic response to vasoconstrictors in hepatorenal syndrome parallels increase in mean arterial pressure: a pooled analysis of clinical trials. *Am J Kidney Dis.* 2011;58(6):928-938.

(either type 1 or 2), evaluation of vasoconstrictor treatment for ≥72 hours, and documentation of serial Cr levels and pre- and posttreatment MAP values. Studies evaluating the role of vasoconstrictors on HRS recurrence were excluded. The primary outcomes were associations between mean daily changes in MAP, serum Cr, urinary output, and plasma renin activity (PRA) on vasoconstrictor treatment.

On vasoconstrictor treatment, an increase in MAP was associated with a decline in serum Cr (rho = −0.76; $P < .001$) but not an increase in urinary output (rho = 0.33; $P = .08$). A decrease in PRA was also associated with decline in serum Cr (rho = 0.70; $P = .001$). When studies were restricted to only include randomized controlled trials, associations between MAP and serum Cr as well as PRA and serum Cr were stronger. In line with evidence of the benefits of vasoconstrictor treatment, AASLD guidelines recommend administration of octreotide and midodrine in the treatment of HRS (Class IIa, Level B) or norepinephrine among ICU patients (Class IIa, Level A).[3]

The patient becomes oliguric and hypotensive and is transferred to the ICU. He receives norepinephrine, which is titrated to goal MAP. His serum Cr drastically improves and urine output increases, and he is weaned off norepinephrine. Over several days, he improves back to his baseline and prepares for discharge home from the hospital. Despite symptom resolution, the patient expresses concern over his overall disease trajectory and prognosis. He mentions the great effort he has put into remaining abstinent from alcohol over the past 5 months with hopes of becoming a liver transplantation candidate in the near future.

What clinical tools can help assess disease trajectory and prioritize organ allocation for liver transplantation?

The Model for End-stage Liver Disease (MELD) score can be used to prioritize organ allocation for liver transplantation. Its use for patients on the transplant list is associated with a survival benefit compared to the former era of organ allocation based on Child-Pugh score.

The MELD score has been evaluated as an alternative to the historical Child-Pugh score for prioritizing liver organ allocation in a large, prospective single-center study comparing transplantation outcomes based on organ allocation during the Child-Pugh (2001-2003) and

MELD (2003-2005) eras.[11] All patients on the liver transplantation list were followed prospectively from March 2003 to March 2005, during which investigators used the MELD score to allocate organs for liver transplantation. Outcomes for this cohort were compared to those of patients listed for transplantation using Child-Pugh scores from March 2001 to March 2003. A total of 563 patients were included, 339 from the MELD era and 224 from the Child-Pugh era. Because the study was based on an existing liver transplantation registry (with placement based on criteria from the American Society of Transplant Physicians and the American Association for the Study of Liver Diseases[12]), no inclusion or exclusion criteria were applied. The primary outcomes included 1-year survival and removal from the transplant waiting list due to death or tumor progression within 6 months.

MELD era patients had higher 1-year survival (84% vs. 72% among Child-Pugh era patients; $P < .05$) and lower rates of removal from the transplant waiting list due to death or tumor progression (10% and 1.2% vs. 16.1% and 4.9% among Child-Pugh era patients, respectively; $P < .05$).

The prognostic benefit of adding hyponatremia to the MELD score was subsequently evaluated in a single-center retrospective cohort study of 308 cirrhotic patients in Spain listed for liver transplantation.[13] Exclusion criteria included hepatocellular carcinoma and noncirrhosis diseases (e.g., acute liver failure). Demographic and clinical variables captured at the time of listing, including serum sodium and calculated MELD score, were evaluated for prognostic value (assessed via area under the receiver operating characteristic curves, AUROC) for the primary outcomes of 3- and 12-month survival after transplant listing.

At 3 months, AUROC for MELD scores and serum sodium were 0.79 (95% CI 0.71-0.86) and 0.83 (95% CI 0.76-0.90), respectively. At 12 months, AUROC for MELD score and serum sodium were 0.77 (95% CI 0.70-0.80) and 0.70 (95% CI 0.60-0.78), respectively. AUROC curves did not differ between MELD score and serum sodium for both outcomes. Caveats include the small sample size from a single-center and retrospective nature of the study.

---

[11]Ravaioli M, et al. Liver transplantation with the Meld system: a prospective study from a single European center. *Am J Transplant.* 2006;6(7):1572-1577.

[12]Wiesner R, et al. Model for end-stage liver disease (MELD) and allocation of donor livers. *Gastroenterology.* 2003;124(1):91-96.

[13]Londoño MC, et al. MELD score and serum sodium in the prediction of survival of patients with cirrhosis awaiting liver transplantation. *Gut.* 2007;56(9):1283-1290.

This study contributed to the 2013 AASLD guidelines that recommend evaluation for liver transplantation based on MELD (score ≥15) or development of overt complications of cirrhosis such as ascites, hepatic encephalopathy, or variceal hemorrhage (Class I, Level A).[14] The United Network for Organ Sharing MELD score calculator is used to prioritize cirrhotic patients for liver transplantation.

> You calculate the patient's MELD score as 22, which correlates with a 3-month mortality rate of 19.6%. You counsel the patient on the importance of continued alcohol abstinence, and he reports motivation to remain abstinent and adhere to his management plan. At discharge, you arrange for an outpatient appointment in the transplant hepatology center.

KEY LEARNING POINTS

1. In cirrhotic patients with SBP and Cr > 1 mg/dL, BUN>30 mg/dL, or total bilirubin >4 mg/dL, albumin infusion is associated with lower risk of renal failure and death.
2. Prophylactic antibiotics should be initiated in cirrhotic patients with either gastrointestinal bleeding, previous SBP, or ascites if ascitic fluid protein <1 g/dL or ascitic fluid protein <1.5 g/dL and Child class C disease.
3. Rifaximin does not appear to be superior to lactulose, which remains the first line option for treating HE.
4. Numerous vasoconstrictors have been shown to be beneficial in increasing MAP among patients with HRS. There is no convincing evidence of one vasoconstrictor being superior to another.
5. The MELD score can be used to prioritize organ allocation for liver transplantation. Its use for patients on the transplant list is associated with a survival benefit compared to the former era of organ allocation based on Child-Pugh score.

---

[14]Martin P, et al. Evaluation for liver transplantation in adults: 2013 practice guideline by the American Association for the Study of Liver Diseases and the American Society of Transplantation. *Hepatology.* 2014;59(3):1144-1165.

CLOSTRIDIOIDES DIFFICILE INFECTION

Courtney Tuegel, MD,
Christopher Kim, MD, MBA

You admit a 50-year-old man with no prior medical history, previously diagnosed left lower extremity cellulitis that has progressed despite oral clindamycin. He is started on intravenous vancomycin and develops four bouts of diarrhea on hospital day 2. In the absence of other explanations or inciting factors, you are concerned for infection with *Clostridioides difficile* (*C. difficile*), formerly known as *Clostridium difficile*.

Which types of commonly used diagnostic tests are available for rapidly detecting *C. difficile* infection (CDI)?

Two-step assays and toxin nucleic acid amplification test polymerase chain reaction (NAAT PCR) are two commonly available, rapid tests for diagnosing CDI.

Despite being the gold standard for diagnosing CDI, toxigenic stool culture is a time-intensive test (e.g., need for special growth medium and follow-up cytotoxic assay, 1-2 day time requirement). Consequently, studies have evaluated test characteristics for more rapid modalities such as two-step assays and toxin NAAT PCR.

A study conducted at two US hospitals within an academic medical center in 2004[1] evaluated the two-step assay, which assesses samples for the presence of *C. difficile* by enzyme immunoassay (EIA) and if pos-

---

[1]Ticehurst JR, et al. Effective detection of toxigenic *Clostridium difficile* by a two-step algorithm including tests for antigen and cytotoxin. *J Clin Microbiol*. 2006;44(3):1145.

itive, progresses to cytotoxicity assay. 266 fecal specimens from hospitalized patients with suspected CDI were sent to the study center and tested via the two-step assay approach. Negative EIA alone had high sensitivity (96%, 95% CI ≥ 79%) and negative predictive value (99.5%, 95% CI ≥ 97.5%) for CDI. These findings support the two-step assay approach and suggest that cytotoxicity assay may not be necessary in EIA-negative samples.

A 2007 observational study done across three hospitals within an academic medical center evaluated the test performance characteristics of toxin NAAT PCR compared to anaerobic culture as a reference gold standard among 618 unformed stool samples.[2] Compared to culture, toxin NAAT PCR had a sensitivity of 94% and specificity of 97%. Caveats include small number of positive CDI cases.

Given the diagnostic effectiveness of both the two-step glutamate dehydrogenase (GDH) EIA/cytotoxic assay and the toxin NAAT PCR, IDSA guidelines support both modalities (weak recommendation, low quality of evidence) as options for testing patients for whom there is clinical suspicion of CDI.[3]

> You send the patient's stool for *C. difficile* toxin NAAT PCR, which returns positive. You diagnose him with CDI and arrange for placement in an isolation room. Your student asks why this is necessary.

What role does exposure to rooms occupied by CDI patients play in the transmission of *C. difficile*?

Exposure in a room occupied by patients with CDI can contribute to the transmission of CDI.

This question was addressed in a 2013 single-site study that evaluated 1770 patients admitted to a 20-bed ICU to determine whether being admitted to a room previously occupied by a patient with a CDI

---

[2]Peterson LR, et al. Detection of toxigenic *Clostridium difficile* in stool samples by real-time polymerase chain reaction for the diagnosis of *C. difficile*-associated diarrhea. *Clin Infect Dis.* 2007;45(9):1152-1160.

[3]McDonald LC et al. Clinical practice guidelines for Clostridium difficile infection in adults and children: 2017 update by the Infectious Diseases Society of America (IDSA) and Society for Healthcare Epidemiology of America (SHEA). *Clin Infect Dis.* 2018;66:987-994.

conferred a higher risk of developing CDI for the new occupant.[4] Acquisition of CDI was measured throughout the duration of patients' ICU stay and in the 30 days after patients transferred out of the ICU. Those diagnosed with CDI before their ICU stay were excluded from the analysis of new CDI acquisition but were included as potential sources of room exposure. CDI was diagnosed by ELISA for *C. difficile* toxins.

After controlling for factors such as antibiotic and proton pump inhibitor use, age, and illness severity, admission to a room whose prior occupant had CDI was associated with greater CDI incidence (HR 2.35, 95% CI 1.21-4.54; $P = .01$). Of note, the study did not control for other medications implicated in CDI risk (e.g., histamine blockers, antimotility agents). Nonetheless, study findings are consistent with IDSA recommendations to use isolation rooms or wards for patients with CDI to limit transmission (strong recommendation, moderate quality of evidence).[5]

> You reassess the patient after he is placed in an isolation room. As you leave, you notice a sign on the door instructing you to wash your hands.

Which modality of hand hygiene is best at eliminating *C. difficile*?

Soap and water hand washing is the preferred modality of hand hygiene for eliminating C. difficile.

Because *C. difficile* endospores can be resistant to elimination with routine hospital antiseptics, this question was addressed in a study of 10 healthy volunteers in Quebec in which modalities of hand hygiene were tested to evaluate their effectiveness for eliminating spores.[6] Six approaches were tested: warm water/plain soap, cold water/plain soap, warm water/antibacterial soap, antiseptic hand wipes, alcohol-based hand rub, and no handwashing. Contamination was achieved by a

---

[4]Shaughnessy MK, et al. Evaluation of hospital room assignment and acquisition of *Clostridium difficile* infection. *Infect Control Hosp Epidemiol.* 2011;32(3):201-206.
[5]See footnote 3.
[6]Oughton MT, et al. Hand hygiene with soap and water is superior to alcohol rub and antiseptic wipes for removal of *Clostridium difficile*. *Infect Control Hosp Epidemiol.* 2009;30:939-944.

"whole-hand protocol," in which 20 mL of a *C. difficile* inoculum was poured into a glove and participants' hands were placed in the glove, and a "surface contamination protocol" in which participants placed both palms on a ceramic tile that was contaminated with *C. difficile*. Participants were not trained in any particular hand washing technique. The outcome of interest was the mean reduction in *C. difficile* colony forming units (CFUs).

In the whole-hand protocol, water (warm or cold) with plain soap led to the greatest mean reductions in *C. difficile* CFUs while alcohol-based hand rub was equivalent to no handwashing. Compared to those from no handwashing, mean reductions were 1.88 $\log_{10}$ cfu/mL (95% CI 1.48-2.28) for cold water with plain soap, 2.14 $\log_{10}$ cfu/mL (95% CI 1.74-2.54) for warm water with plain soap, and 0.06 (95% CI −0.34 to 0.45) for alcohol-based hand rub (no *P*-values reported). In the surface contamination protocol, both warm water with plain soap (26.63 log10 cfu/mL, 95% CI 24.48-28.77) and cold water with plain soap (26.56 log10 cfu/mL, 95% CI 24.42-28.71) yielded greater reductions in C. difficile CFUs compared to alcohol-based hand rub (no p-values reported).

This evidence about the comparative benefits of soap and water is consistent with IDSA recommendations to preferentially use water with soap over alcohol-based hand hygiene in CDI outbreak settings (strong recommendation, moderate quality of evidence for hand hygiene; weak recommendation, low quality of evidence for preferential water and soap) and use either soap and water or alcohol-based hand hygiene in routine or endemic settings (strong recommendation, moderate quality of evidence).[7]

Unfortunately, the patient's symptoms continue. You diagnose him with nonfulminant CDI and consider treatment options.

What are preferred treatment strategies for first episodes of nonfulminant CDI?

For first episodes of nonfulminant CDI, vancomycin or fidaxomicin is the preferred agent. Metronidazole may be used if vancomycin or fidaxomicin is not available.

---

[7]See footnote 3.

This question was addressed in a 2017 retrospective cohort study of 10,137 patients (both inpatients and outpatients) in the VA health system.[8] Patients with incident CDI treated with oral vancomycin versus oral metronidazole were compared with the primary outcomes of all-cause 30-day mortality and recurrent CDI (defined as repeat positive lab test for CDI >14 days but <56 days from initial diagnosis). Outcomes were evaluated for patients with mild to moderate CDI and severe CDI (defined as leukocytosis >15,000 white blood cells/uL or elevated Cr 1.5 times baseline within 4 days of CDI diagnosis). Patients were excluded if they received both antibiotics within 2 days of CDI diagnosis or if they did not receive either of the study antibiotic for treatment. Importantly, authors only included each individual's first case of CDI *that met study eligibility criteria*, whether it was the patient's first or recurrent episode of CDI.

Mortality was lower in the vancomycin group (8.6% vs. 10.6% in the metronidazole group, RR 0.86, 95% CI 0.74-0.98; *P* = .01), primarily from a 4.5% absolute risk reduction (ARR) among patients with severe CDI (15.3% vs. 19.8% in the metronidazole group, RR 0.79, 95% CI 0.65-0.97; *P* = .01). There was no difference in recurrence rate of CDI between the two treatment groups (RR 0.98, 95% CI 0.87-1.10; no *P*-value reported).

A multicenter, double-blinded, randomized clinical trial at 67 North American sites randomized 629 patients (both inpatients and outpatients) with CDI to 10 days of oral vancomycin (125 mg four times daily) versus oral fidaxomicin (200 mg twice daily).[9] Patients with fulminant CDI, previous exposure to fidaxomicin, and >1 recurrence of CDI in the prior 3 months were excluded. The primary outcome was rate of clinical cure (symptom resolution without need for additional treatment 2 days after completing therapy), and secondary outcomes included recurrence (assessed weekly for 28 days via diarrhea log and a positive stool toxin result).

The groups did not differ with respect to clinical cure (88.2% in fidaxomicin group vs. 85.8% in the vancomycin group; *P*-value not reported). Treatment with fidaxomicin resulted in less recurrence (15.4% vs. 25.3% in the vancomycin group, 95% CI -16.6--2.9; *P* = .005). The recurrence reduction was predominantly seen among less virulent C.

[8]Stevens VW, et al. Comparative effectiveness of vancomycin and metronidazole for the prevention of recurrence and death in patients with *Clostridium difficile* infection. *JAMA Intern Med.* 2017.

[9]Louie TJ, et al. Fidaxomicin versus vancomycin for *Clostridium difficile* infection. *N Engl J Med.* 2011;364:422-431.

difficile strains. Study caveats include lack of information about certain CDI risk factors, such as proton pump inhibitor use.

In line with these studies, IDSA guidelines recommend either vancomycin or fidaxomicin for initial nonfulminant CDI regardless of disease severity. Metronidazole is recommended only if vancomycin or fidaxomicin is not available (strong recommendation, high quality of evidence).[10]

You initiate oral vancomycin, and the patient's condition improves. The next day, another patient is admitted to your service with recurrent CDI. In reviewing her chart, you note that she has been treated for CDI a total of three times in the 6 months since her first diagnosis. You consider whether fecal microbiota transplantation (FMT) would be appropriate, given her recurrent infections.

What is the role of FMT in treating recurrent CDI?

Healthy gut flora repopulation through FMT should be considered for patients with multiple CDI recurrences.

The role of FMT—transplant of healthy donor feces into patients with CDI—was evaluated in an open-label randomized clinical trial[11] including 43 adult patients who had ≥1 relapse of CDI. Patients were randomized to one of three arms: oral vancomycin alone for 14 days, vancomycin for 14 days followed by nasoduodenal FMT, or vancomycin for 14 days followed by nasoduodenal bowel lavage. ICU and immunocompromised patients and those using antibiotics for non-CDI reasons at baseline were excluded. The primary outcome was cure (diarrhea explainable by other etiologies or no diarrhea, plus three consecutive negative *C. difficile* stool toxin tests) without relapse of CDI at 10 weeks after start of therapy.

At interim analysis, 13/16 (81%) patients receiving FMT were cured without relapse compared to 4/13 (31%) patients receiving vancomycin alone and 3/13 patients (23%) receiving vancomycin with bowel lavage ($P < .001$). Further, the 3 patients who had recurrence of their CDI in the FMT group were administered a second infusion of FMT from

---

[10]See footnote 3.
[11]van Nood E, et al. Duodenal infusion of donor feces for recurrent *Clostridium difficile*. *N Engl J Med.* 2013;368:407-415.

a different healthy donor, and 2/3 were cured of their CDI without relapse. Based on these results, the trial was stopped early.

In another randomized trial evaluating FMT,[12] 46 patients who had ≥3 recurrent CDIs and were not cured despite tapered or pulsed vancomycin were randomized to vancomycin therapy followed by either autologous or donor FMT. Exclusion criteria included age >75 years, immunocompromised state, previous FMT, inflammatory bowel disease, and irritable bowel syndrome. The primary outcome was rate of clinical cure (defined by <3 stools per day) at 8 weeks after FMT.

The primary outcome occurred more frequently in the donor FMT group (91% vs. 63%, $P = .042$). The nine patients with recurrence of their CDI in the autologous FMT group subsequently received FMT from a donor, and all nine then achieved cure. Caveats include lack of data on CDI severity prior to FMT.

Nonetheless, in agreement with this evidence, IDSA guidelines strongly recommend FMT in patients with multiple recurrences of CDI despite appropriate antibiotics (strong recommendation, moderate quality of evidence).[13]

> You consult gastroenterology to consider FMT for her recurrent CDI.

KEY LEARNING POINTS

1. Two-step assays and toxin NAAT PCR are two commonly available, rapid tests for diagnosing CDI.
2. Exposure in a room occupied by patients with CDI can contribute to the transmission of CDI.
3. Soap and water hand washing is the preferred modality of hand hygiene for eliminating *C. difficile*.
4. For first episodes of nonfulminant CDI, vancomycin or fidaxomicin is the preferred agent. Metronidazole may be used if vancomycin or fidaxomicin is not available.
5. Healthy gut flora repopulation through FMT should be considered for patients with multiple CDI recurrences.

---

[12]Kelly CR, et al. Effect of fecal microbiota transplantation on recurrence in multiply recurrent Clostridium difficile infection: a randomized trial. *Ann Intern Med*. 2016;165:609-616.
[13]See footnote 3.

23 VENTRICULAR TACHYCARDIA

Christopher P. Kovach, MD, MSc,
Mala M. Sanchez, MD

You admit a 68-year-old woman with atrial fibrillation, hypertension, and hyperlipidemia who presented with 15- to 30-second episodes of lightheadedness and palpitations. She reports weight gain and leg swelling after a recent holiday celebration with family, after which she has not been able to sleep without propping herself with pillows. Shortly after admission, you are paged that she is experiencing active palpitations. At the bedside, you find the patient awake and without acute distress. She is tachycardic with heart rate in the 170s and a normal blood pressure.

Her telemetry rhythm strip demonstrates the following wide-complex tachycardia (WCT):

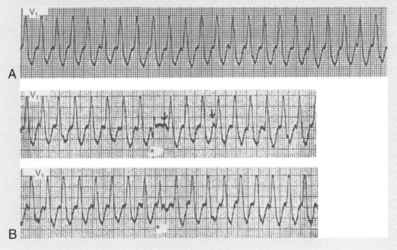

(continued)

You compare this tracing to the patient's baseline ECG (shown below) and weigh whether the patient's current WCT is more consistent with sustained monomorphic ventricular tachycardia (hereafter stable VT) or supraventricular tachycardia (SVT) with aberrancy.

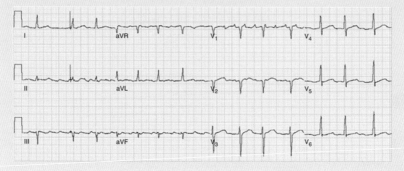

How can VT and SVT with aberrancy be distinguished by ECG?

Algorithmic ECG interpretation approaches can be used to differentiate VT from SVT with aberrancy. In particular, the presence of atrioventricular (AV) dissociation *or* precordial QRS concordance *or* northwest QRS axis (>270°) by ECG is nearly 100% predictive of VT.

In a narrative review,[1] authors discussed selected studies published over a period of 50 years that focused on deriving and/or validating the ability of ECG findings to predict VT. Stratifying their findings by QRS morphology, the authors reported positive predictive value (PPV) for a range of ECG findings (Table 23.1). Of these, they found that the presence of AV dissociation, QRS concordance in the precordial leads, and extreme "northwest" QRS axis (i.e., >270°) were the most suggestive of VT in both left and right bundle branch QRS morphologies. Three ECG findings that suggest AV dissociation are (1) QRS complexes occurring more rapidly than, and independently of, P waves, (2) the presence of intermittent normal, nonwide QRS complexes interrupting the WCT (known as "capture beats"), and (3) the presence of hybrid atrial/ventricular complexes interrupting the WCT (known as "fusion beats").

---

[1]Garner JB, Miller JM. Wide complex tachycardia – ventricular tachycardia or not ventricular tachycardia, that remains the question. *Arrhythm Electrophysiol Rev.* 2013;2(1):23-29.

TABLE 23.1

PPV of Specific ECG Criteria for the Identification of VT

	LBBB/RBBB Morphology
AV dissociation	100%
Precordial concordance	89%-90%
Northwest axis	95%-96%
	LBBB morphology
QRS width >160 ms	98%-99%
Right axis deviation	87%-96%
	RBBB morphology
RSR' in V1 (left peak > right peak)	100%
Left axis deviation	88%-96%
QRS width >140 ms	89%

AV, atrioventricular; LBBB, left bundle branch block; RBBB, right bundle branch block; VT, ventricular tachycardia.

Adapted from Garner JB, Miller JM. Wide complex tachycardia – ventricular tachycardia or not ventricular tachycardia, that remains the question. *Arrhythm Electrophysiol Rev.* 2013;2(1):23-29.

Multiple algorithms for interpreting ECG findings and differentiating between VT and SVT with aberrancy have been established. A retrospective analysis[2] of 260 WCTs evaluated the performance characteristics of the Brugada, Bayesian, Griffith, lead aVR, and lead II R-wave peak time algorithms in a sample of 204 patients. ECGs from unselected, consecutive patients were analyzed using algorithms by a blinded cardiologist and cardiac electrophysiologist. Ultimate diagnoses were confirmed by the study team via either electrophysiology (EP) study, intracardiac ECG from an implanted device, or subsequent ECGs. The algorithms were found to have similarly moderate diagnostic accuracy for VT (i.e., arrived at the correct diagnosis approximately 69%-77% of the time). The Brugada algorithm was found to have superior accuracy compared to R-wave peak time ($P = .04$).

---

[2]Jastrzebski M, et al. Comparison of five electrocardiographic methods for differentiation of wide QRS-complex tachycardias. *Europace.* 2012;14(8):1165-1171.

Upon recheck, her heart rate continues to be elevated in the 160s-170s with normal blood pressure. Based on these vital signs and her ECG and rhythm strip findings, which show AV dissociation and fusion beats, you conclude that she is currently in stable VT and consider pharmacologic options for terminating the rhythm.

Which antiarrhythmic drugs can be used to terminate stable VT?

Several medications have efficacy for terminating stable VT, including amiodarone, lidocaine, and procainamide. In particular, evidence supports the effectiveness of procainamide.

This question was addressed in a 2013 systematic review[3] that screened 574 studies and ultimately identified 5 high-quality studies (3 prospective, 2 retrospective) comparing the effect of IV antiarrhythmics on stable VT. Studies measuring the suppressive effect of IV drugs on electrophysiologic inducibility of VT were excluded. The authors determined that procainamide was superior to lidocaine (RR 2.2, 95% CI 1.2-4.0; P-value not reported; number needed to treat [NNT] 2.5) but that amiodarone and procainamide were equivalent (RR 4.3, 95% CI 0.8-23.6; NNT 3.0). A major study caveat was limited available evidence.

A subsequent multicenter randomized-controlled trial, PROCAMIO,[4] compared the efficacy of procainamide and amiodarone in terminating stable VT. Seventy-four patients with presumed stable VT (based on the presence of WCT on ECG and lack of response to vagal maneuvers or adenosine) were randomized to IV procainamide versus IV amiodarone. The primary efficacy outcome was the proportion of patients whose WCT terminated within 40 minutes of drug administration, while the primary safety outcome was incidence of major adverse cardiac events (e.g., hypotension, pulmonary edema) within 40 minutes of drug administration.

---

[3]deSouza IS, et al. Antidysrhythmic drug therapy for the termination of stable, monomorphic ventricular tachycardia: a systematic review. *Emerg Med J.* 2015;32:161-167.

[4]Ortiz M, et al; PROCAMIO Study Investigators. Randomized comparison of intravenous procainamide vs. intravenous amiodarone for the acute treatment of tolerated wide QRS tachycardia: the PROCAMIO study. *Eur Heart J.* 2017;38(17):1329-1335.

More patients in the procainamide group had VT terminated within 40 minutes (67% vs. 38%, OR 3.3, 95% CI 1.2-9.3; P = .03). Adverse cardiac events occurred in more patients from the amiodarone group (41% vs. 9%, OR 0.1, 95% CI 0.03-0.6; P = .006). In the 24 hours after drug administration, amiodarone was also more likely to cause hypotension while procainamide was more likely to be associated with QT prolongation. Study caveats include potential underpowering; recruitment was stopped due to low event rate and inability to reach the preplanned enrollment thresholds after 6 years.

Studies have also demonstrated the comparative efficacy of procainamide over lidocaine in acute termination of stable VT. A randomized-controlled trial[5] demonstrated that among 29 patients randomized to receive either IV procainamide or lidocaine, more patients in the procainamide group had their VT terminated (80% vs. 21%; P < .01). Study caveats include the exclusion of patients with severe heart failure, acute myocardial infarction (MI), or significant liver or kidney disorders. The 2017 American Heart Association (AHA)/American College of Cardiology (ACC)/Heart Rhythm Society (HRS) guidelines[6] incorporate the findings of the above studies, noting the potential usefulness of procainamide in terminating hemodynamically stable VT (class IIa, LOE [level of evidence] A) alongside amiodarone as another agent to be considered (class IIb, LOE B-R).

> You administer IV procainamide to the patient, who responds and converts to sinus rhythm. A repeat ECG shows no evidence of acute ischemia. She is monitored overnight on telemetry without incident. On rounds the next morning, the patient states she has never had this type of tachycardia before and inquires about any required additional testing.

---

[5]Gorgels AP, et al. Comparison of procainamide and lidocaine in terminating sustained monomorphic ventricular tachycardia. *Am J Cardiol.* 1996;78(1):43-46.
[6]Al-Khatib SM, et al. 2017 AHA/ACC/HRS guideline for management of patients with ventricular arrhythmias and the prevention of sudden cardiac death. *J Am Coll Cardiol.* 2018;72:e91-e220.

What is the role of cardiac imaging in the evaluation of newly diagnosed VT?

Imaging should be obtained to assess left ventricular ejection fraction (LVEF), given that decreased LVEF is a strong predictor of sudden cardiac death (SCD) and mortality. Decreased LVEF is also one of the indications for implantable cardiac defibrillator (ICD) placement.

This issue was addressed in a secondary analysis of patients from VALIANT,[7] a randomized-controlled trial in which 14,703 patients with decreased LVEF (<40%) or clinical or radiologic evidence of heart failure after MI were randomized to treatment with valsartan, captopril, or both. To assess incidence and timing of SCD or cardiac arrest among these patients, researchers evaluated these outcomes over time for patients stratified by LVEF: >40%, 31% to 40%, and ≤30%. Median follow-up was 25 months.

Patients with LVEF ≤30% had a higher incidence of SCD (10%) compared to those with LVEF 31% to 40% (6%) or LVEF >40% (5%) over the study period. Treating LVEF as a continuous variable demonstrated that a 5% decrease in LVEF was associated with a 21% increase in SCD or cardiac arrest (HR 1.21, 95% CI 1.10-1.30; P-value not reported) within the first 30 days after MI. Caveats include the fact that the incidence of SCD or cardiac arrest was not assessed in patients without decreased LVEF or clinical/radiographic heart failure after MI. Nonetheless, the AHA/ACC/HRS guidelines[5] recommend an assessment of global and regional myocardial function in patients with known or suspected ventricular arrhythmias (class I, LOE B).

A transthoracic echocardiogram (TTE) reveals decreased LVEF with regional wall motion abnormalities, suggestive of a prior MI. Additional evaluation does not reveal reversible causes of VT. You are therefore suspicious for underlying ischemic heart disease and pursue left heart catheterization, which confirms multivessel disease. You begin guideline-directed medical therapy and consider other interventions that can reduce her risk of such events.

---

[7]Solomon SD, et al. Sudden death in patients with myocardial infarction and left ventricular dysfunction, heart failure, or both. *N Engl J Med.* 2005;352(25):2581-2588.

What are nonpharmacologic options for preventing SCD in patients with VT?

An ICD should be placed for secondary prevention of SCD in patients with structural heart disease who survive VT not due to a reversible cause.

This question was addressed through three randomized-controlled trials—AVID, CASH, and CIDS—that evaluated the role of ICDs versus medical therapy in secondary prevention of SCD. Results from these studies were subsequently pooled in a preplanned meta-analysis.[8] Published in 2000, the meta-analysis included a total of 1866 patients with an average LVEF of 34% who had experienced either ventricular fibrillation, symptomatic VT, or syncope with a subsequent diagnosis of VT. 96% of patients in the pooled database had some form of structural heart disease. Compared to amiodarone, ICD therapy was associated with lower all-cause mortality (HR 0.73, 95% CI 0.60-0.87; $P < .001$) and death from arrhythmia (HR 0.49, 95% CI 0.36-0.67; $P < .001$).

Accordingly, AHA/ACC/HRS guidelines[5] recommend that patients with ischemic heart disease or other cardiomyopathy who have experienced sustained VT have an ICD placed for secondary prevention (class I, LOE B).

The patient undergoes successful ICD placement and is discharged home off of antiarrhythmic medications. However, she returns to the ED and is readmitted a few weeks later after ICD shocks at home. Device interrogation reveals that these were appropriate shocks given for recurrent VT.

What therapies can reduce shocks and admissions for patients with VT after ICD?

Antiarrhythmic medications such as beta-blockers and amiodarone can improve quality of life and reduce appropriate or inappropriate ICD shocks in patients with VT.

---

[8]Connolly SJ, et al. Meta-analysis of the implantable cardioverter defibrillator secondary prevention trials. AVID, CASH, and CIDS studies. Antiarrhythmics vs implantable defibrillator study. Cardiac arrest study Hamburg. Canadian implantable defibrillator study. *Eur Heart J.* 2000;21(24):2071-2078.

Given the negative impact that both appropriate and inappropriate ICD shocks can have on patients, the OPTIC study[9] evaluated the role of medications in reducing the rate of these shocks among patients with ICDs. OPTIC was a multinational randomized-controlled trial in which 412 patients with recent ICDs placed for secondary prevention of VT or VF were randomized to receive 1 year of either sotalol alone, beta-blocker alone, or combination therapy with amiodarone and a beta-blocker. Patients were included if they had LVEF <40% and ICD placement within the preceding 21 days for stable VT, VF, or cardiac arrest. Patients with New York Heart Association (NYHA) class IV heart failure symptoms were excluded. The primary outcome was ICD shock for any reason. Other outcomes included adverse pulmonary events, adverse thyroid events, and symptomatic bradycardia.

Combination therapy reduced the risk of ICD shock compared to sotalol alone (HR 0.43, 95% CI 0.22-0.85; $P = .02$) and beta-blocker alone (HR 0.27, 95% CI 0.14-0.52, $P < .001$). However, symptomatic bradycardia and adverse pulmonary and thyroid events were more common in the combination therapy group compared to the sotalol-alone and beta-blocker-alone groups. Study limitations included a low event rate of ICD shocks in the study population and lack of a formal quality-of-life outcome assessment.

> After discussing risks and benefits, the patient agrees to initiate amiodarone and a beta-blocker. In preparation for discharge home, she asks you if there are treatment options if she continues to experience ICD shocks for VT despite being on these medications.

What therapies can benefit patients with VT who continue to experience recurrent VT despite ICD and antiarrhythmic therapy?

Ablation therapy can be beneficial in patients with prior MI who have recurrent VT despite ICD placement and antiarrhythmic therapy.

This issue was explored in the VANISH trial,[10] which randomized 259 patients to catheter ablation with continuation of antiarrhythmic

---

[9]Connolly SJ, et al. Comparison of beta-blockers, amiodarone plus beta-blockers, or sotalol for prevention of shocks from implantable cardioverter defibrillators: the OPTIC Study: a randomized trial. *J Am Med Assoc.* 2006;295:165-171.

[10]Sapp JL, et al. Ventricular tachycardia ablation versus escalation of antiarrhythmic drugs. *New Engl J Med.* 2016;375(2):111-121.

medications versus escalation of antiarrhythmic medication therapy (i.e., escalated therapy). Patients were eligible for inclusion if they had suffered a MI, undergone ICD placement, and had an episode of VT during treatment with a class I or class III antiarrhythmic drug during the preceding 6 months. Patients with an active acute coronary syndrome, recent ST-elevation myocardial infarction (STEMI), or recent coronary revascularization were excluded. The primary outcome was a composite of death, ≥3 documented episodes of VT within 24 hours, or appropriate ICD shock.

Compared to escalated therapy, ablation was associated with a lower rate of the primary outcome (HR 0.72, 95% CI 0.53-0.98; *P* = .04). A study caveat is that the benefit observed with respect to the primary outcome was largely driven by reduction in the rate of VT storm and ICD shocks rather than mortality. AHA/ACC/HRS guidelines[5] recommend consideration of ablation therapy in patients with prior MI and recurrent episodes of stable VT who are intolerant of amiodarone (class I, LOE B-R) or other antiarrhythmic therapy (class I, LOE B-NR).

KEY LEARNING POINTS

1. Algorithmic ECG interpretation approaches can be used to differentiate VT from SVT with aberrancy. In particular, the presence of AV dissociation *or* precordial QRS concordance *or* northwest QRS axis (>270°) by ECG is nearly 100% predictive of VT.

2. Several medications have efficacy for terminating stable VT, including amiodarone, lidocaine, and procainamide. In particular, evidence supports the effectiveness of procainamide.

3. Cardiac imaging should be obtained to assess LVEF given that decreased LVEF is a strong predictor of SCD and mortality. Decreased LVEF is also one of the indications for ICD placement.

4. An ICD should be placed for secondary prevention of SCD in patients with structural heart disease who survive VT not due to a reversible cause.

5. Antiarrhythmic medications such as beta-blockers and amiodarone can improve quality of life and reduce appropriate or inappropriate ICD shocks in patients with VT.

6. Ablation therapy can be beneficial in patients with prior MI who have recurrent VT despite ICD placement and antiarrhythmic therapy.

PERIOPERATIVE MEDICINE

Divya Gollapudi, MD

A 70 year-old man with history of coronary artery disease with prior stent placement, atrial fibrillation, hypertension, and type 2 diabetes mellitus is admitted with a right-displaced femur fracture after a ground level fall. He denies chest pain, dyspnea, or presyncope. His troponin is negative, and ECG demonstrates atrial fibrillation without ST-T changes. The patient recently underwent a dobutamine stress echocardiogram for evaluation of chronic stable dyspnea on exertion, which demonstrated a small inferolateral wall motion abnormality with stress. You consider if this patient requires a delay in surgery to potentially undergo further evaluation of his coronary artery disease prior to surgery.

What is the role of coronary revascularization in reducing perioperative cardiac complications for patients with stable coronary artery disease?

Coronary revascularization is not recommended for patients with stable coronary artery disease prior to noncardiac surgery exclusively to decrease perioperative cardiac events.

This question was considered in the Coronary Artery Revascularization Prophylaxis (CARP) trial,[1] which studied patients with stable coronary artery disease undergoing elective vascular surgery. In CARP, 5859 patients considered at increased risk for

---

[1]McFalls EO, et al. Coronary-artery revascularization before elective major vascular surgery. *N Engl J Med.* 2004;351(27):2795-2804.

perioperative cardiac complications (as determined by a cardiologist) underwent coronary angiogram. Of these, the 510 with at least 70% stenosis in a coronary vessel were subsequently randomized to either receive or not receive preoperative revascularization with percutaneous coronary intervention or coronary artery bypass grafting prior to surgery (for an expanding abdominal aortic aneurysm or severe symptoms of arterial occlusive disease of the legs). Exclusion criteria included left main disease, left ventricular ejection fraction <20%, or severe aortic stenosis, and prior revascularization without evidence of recurrent ischemia. The primary outcome was long-term mortality (as ascertained via follow-up and longitudinal database), and secondary outcomes included 30-day mortality and myocardial infarction (MI).

The median time from randomization to vascular surgery was longer among those receiving preoperative revascularization (54 vs. 18 days among not receiving revascularization, $P < .001$). After a median of 2.7 years, there was no difference in long-term mortality (22% vs. 23%, RR 0.98, 95% CI 0.70-1.37; $P = .92$). There was also no difference in 30-day postoperative death or MI. One caveat relates to the fact that the majority of patients in both groups were on medical therapy with beta-blockers, aspirin, and/or statins preoperatively, which could have itself provided perioperative cardiac protection and diminished the differences in long-term mortality between the study groups. A subsequently published analysis[2] of the randomized and nonrandomized (excluded) patients of the initial CARP trial cohort revealed that patients with left main coronary disease had improved survival with preoperative coronary revascularization (RR = 0.84 vs. 0.52 among patients without perioperative revascularization; $P < .01$).

Due to the lack of compelling evidence for coronary vascular intervention preoperatively in this high-risk population, the 2014 ACCAHA guidelines on perioperative cardiac evaluation[3] recommend that preoperative coronary revascularization be reserved only for unstable coronary syndromes or circumstances for which practice guidelines for

[2]Garcia S, et al. Usefulness of revascularization of patients with multivessel coronary artery disease before elective vascular surgery for abdominal aortic and peripheral occlusive disease. *Am J Cardiol.* 2008;102:809-813.

[3]Fleisher LA, et al. 2014 ACC/AHA guideline on perioperative cardiovascular evaluation and management of patients undergoing noncardiac surgery: executive summary: a report of the American College of Cardiology/American Heart Association Task Force on Practice Guidelines. *Circulation.* 2014;130(24):2215-2245.

revascularization already exist, such as left main disease (class I recommendation, level C evidence). This recommendation, although based on data from elective vascular surgery patients, has been broadly applied to noncardiac surgeries.

The patient is scheduled for operative repair of his femur fracture with orthopedic surgery for the next day. His outpatient medication list includes warfarin, amlodipine, aspirin, diltiazem, atorvastatin, and metformin. You notice that his medication list does not include a β-blocker, and the patient confirms that he is not currently taking a β-blocker. Given his upcoming surgery and known coronary artery disease, you consider if a β-blocker should be initiated tonight.

What are the risks and benefits of perioperative β-blocker therapy?

Although perioperative β-blocker therapy can reduce risk of perioperative MI, initiation of beta-blocker therapy within 1 day of surgery or in patients considered low risk for perioperative cardiac complications can increase perioperative stroke and mortality.

This question was addressed in a 2014 systematic review[4] that compared perioperative β-blocker therapy with placebo during noncardiac surgery. The review included 17 studies (16 randomized controlled trials, 1 cohort study) and evaluated several cardiac outcomes, including perioperative MI, all-cause mortality, and stroke. The authors reported that among the randomized controlled trials, preoperative initiation of β-blockers decreased nonfatal MI (RR 0.68, 95% CI 0.57-0.81; $P < .001$) and increased nonfatal stroke (RR 1.79; 95% CI 1.09-2.95; $P = .02$), hypotension (RR 1.47; 95% CI 1.34-1.60; $P < .001$), and bradycardia (RR 2.61; 95% CI 2.18-3.12; $P < .001$). All-cause mortality appeared similar between β-blocker and no-β-blocker therapy (RR 0.96; 95% CI 0.62-1.47; $P = .633$).

---

[4]Wijeysundera DN, et al. Perioperative beta-blockade in noncardiac surgery: a systematic review for the 2014 ACC/AHA guideline on perioperative cardiovascular evaluation and management of patients undergoing noncardiac surgery: a report of the American College of Cardiology/American Heart Association Task Force on Practice Guidelines. *Circulation.* 2014;130:2246-2264.

One caveat of this systematic review is that the cumulative data included data from the DECREASE-I[5] and DECREASE-IV[6] trials, the results of which have been seriously questioned due to concerns of scientific misconduct. DECREASE-I and DECREASE-IV were the only trials to demonstrate a mortality benefit of perioperative β-blocker therapy and the only trials included in the meta-analysis to start β-blockers >1 day prior to noncardiac surgery. After excluding these trials, the remaining studies demonstrated an *increase* in all-cause mortality with β-blocker therapy (RR 1.30, 95% CI 1.03-1.64; P = .03), suggesting that initiating β-blockers within 1 day of surgery can cause substantial harm.

A separate, older retrospective cohort study[7] evaluated perioperative β-blocker therapy in routine clinical practice among 663,635 patients who underwent noncardiac surgery at 329 US hospitals. Patients who received β-blockers during the first 2 days of hospitalization (18% of the study cohort) were propensity-matched with nonrecipients with similar baseline characteristics, which included demographics, cardiac comorbidities, concomitant therapy with other cardiac medications (i.e., statins, angiotensin-converting enzyme inhibitors/angiotensin receptor blockers, antiplatelet agents), Revised Cardiac Risk Index (RCRI) score, and type of surgery. β-blocker therapy was associated with a significant reduction in in-hospital mortality among the patients with RCRI scores of 3 (OR 0.71, 95% CI 0.56-0.91; no P-value reported) and ≥ 4 (OR 0.58, 95% CI 0.42-0.76; no P-value reported). Conversely, in-hospital mortality was higher among the lowest-risk patients with RCRI scores of 0 (OR 1.43, 95% CI 1.29-1.58) and 1 (1.13 95% CI 0.99-1.30) who received β-blockers. The small mortality benefit of β-blockers in patients with RCRI scores of 2 was not statistically significant.

Based on the above evidence, the 2014 ACC/AHA perioperative cardiac evaluation guidelines[3] recommend consideration of perioperative β-blocker therapy for patients with intermediate- or high-risk myocardial ischemia on cardiac testing (class IIb recommendation,

[5]Poldermans D, et al. The effect of bisoprolol on perioperative mortality and myocardial infarction in high-risk patients undergoing vascular surgery. Dutch Echocardiographic Cardiac Risk Evaluation Applying Stress Echocardiography Study Group. *N Engl J Med*. 1999;341:1789-1794.

[6]Dunkelgrun M, et al. Bisoprolol and fluvastatin for the reduction of perioperative cardiac mortality and myocardial infarction in intermediate-risk patients undergoing noncardiovascular surgery: a randomized controlled trial (DECREASE-IV). *Ann Surg*. 2009;249:921-926.

[7]Lindenauer PK, et al. Perioperative beta-blocker therapy and mortality after major noncardiac surgery. *N Engl J Med*. 2005;353(4):349-361.

level C evidence), RCRI score ≥ 3 (class IIb recommendation, level B evidence), or compelling long-term indication (class IIB recommendation, level B evidence). The guidelines, however, recommend against initiating β-blockers <1 day prior to surgery (class III recommendation, level B evidence).

> The patient is not started on a β-blocker due to the timing of surgery. While performing his medication reconciliation, you also consider whether to continue his aspirin perioperatively.

What are the risks and benefits of continuing aspirin therapy perioperatively in patients undergoing noncardiac surgery?

The perioperative management of aspirin in patients undergoing noncardiac surgery remains controversial. Data suggest that perioperative aspirin therapy is associated with higher rates of major bleeding, with no significant reduction in rate of all-cause mortality and nonfatal MI. There may be cardiac morbidity and mortality benefit in patients with prior percutaneous coronary intervention.

This clinical question was studied in the 2014 POISE-2 (Perioperative Ischemic Evaluation 2)[8] trial, which was a 2 × 2 factorial trial investigating perioperative aspirin and clonidine therapy. The aspirin arm of this trial randomized 10,010 patients undergoing noncardiac surgery to aspirin or placebo. Patients undergoing carotid endarterectomy and those with recent stents (bare metal stent within the previous 6 weeks, drug-eluting stent within the previous year) were excluded. Aspirin at a dose of 200 mg or placebo was administered immediately prior to surgery. Among patients who had not been on aspirin previously, the study drug was continued for 30 days postoperatively. Patients already on an aspirin regimen at baseline had their medication stopped an average of 1 week prior to surgery and continued the study drug for 7 days postoperatively, after which they resumed their home aspirin regimen. The primary outcome was a composite of death or nonfatal MI at 30 days, and major bleeding was one of several safety outcomes.

The primary outcome occurred at the same rate in aspirin and placebo groups (7.0% vs. 7.1%, HR 0.99, 95% CI 0.86-1.15; *P* = .92). This

---

[8]Devereaux PJ, et al. Aspirin in patients undergoing noncardiac surgery. *N Engl J Med.* 2014;370(16):1494-1503.

finding was similar between patients who were taking aspirin prior to the surgery and those who were not. Aspirin increased the risk of major bleeding as compared with placebo (4.6% vs. 3.8%, HR 1.23, 95% CI 1.01-1.49; $P = .04$). The most common sites of bleeding were the surgical site (78.3%) and gastrointestinal tract (9.3%).

It is important to note that patients undergoing major vascular surgery, patients with coronary artery disease, and patients with coronary stents represented a small proportion of the total study cohort. The study investigators subsequently published a nonprespecified subgroup analysis of patients with prior percutaneous coronary intervention originally included in the POISE-2 trial.[9] In patients with prior percutaneous coronary intervention, aspirin reduced the risk of the primary outcome (HR 0.50, 95% CI 0.26-0.95; $P = .036$), as well as MI (HR 0.44, 95% CI 0.22-0.87; $P = .021$). Notably, the median time from stent placement to noncardiac surgery was 64.0 months.

The 2014 ACC/AHA perioperative guidelines[3] state that the risks of bleeding versus ischemic events should be considered in determining the appropriateness of continuing aspirin in patients without previous coronary stenting who are undergoing elective noncardiac surgery (class IIb recommendation, level B evidence).

> The patient is continued on low-dose aspirin and undergoes his surgery without immediate complication. He is started on subcutaneous enoxaparin for venous thromboembolism prophylaxis, and the pharmacist asks you if the patient requires bridging anticoagulation for his atrial fibrillation.

Which patients with atrial fibrillation on anticoagulation can safely avoid perioperative bridging anticoagulation?

Patients with atrial fibrillation who are on warfarin and considered low risk for stroke can avoid perioperative bridging anticoagulation, which increases bleeding risk without significantly reducing risk of thromboembolism.

---

[9]Graham MM, et al. Aspirin in patients with previous percutaneous coronary intervention undergoing noncardiac surgery. *Ann Intern Med.* 2018;168(4):237-244.

This question was evaluated in the BRIDGE trial,[10] a multicenter, double-blind, randomized, placebo-controlled noninferiority trial evaluating the role of perioperative bridge anticoagulation for elective operations. In BRIDGE, 1884 adult patients with chronic atrial fibrillation/chronic atrial fibrillation or flutter on warfarin discontinued their anticoagulant 5 days prior to surgery and were then randomized to either perioperative bridging with low-molecular-weight heparin (dalteparin) versus placebo. Warfarin was restarted postoperatively per the same protocol in both groups. Participants were anticoagulated for ≥3 months prior to procedure and had a mean $CHADS_2$ score of 2.3. Exclusion criteria included mechanical heart valves, stroke or transient ischemic attack (TIA) within 6 weeks, and planned cardiac, spinal, and neurological surgeries. Coprimary outcomes were arterial thromboembolism (stroke, TIA, systemic embolism) and major bleeding within 30 days. Secondary outcomes were MI, deep vein thrombosis, pulmonary embolism, death, and minor bleeding.

The incidence of arterial thromboembolism was 0.3% in the perioperative bridging group and 0.4% in the no-bridging group (risk difference 0.1%, 95% CI −0.6 to 0.8; $P = .01$ for the prespecified noninferiority margin). Patients who received perioperative bridging had a higher rate of major bleeding as compared to those who did not (3.2% vs. 1.3%, RR 0.41; 95% CI 0.20-0.78; $P = .005$ for superiority). No bridging was superior with regard to minor bleeding (12% vs. 20%; $P < .001$) but not for other secondary outcomes. The major caveat of BRIDGE is that the majority of patients had $CHADS_2$ scores <4, and therefore these results may not be applicable to patients with higher thromboembolic risk.

Based on BRIDGE trial and additional observational studies, the 2017 ACC Expert Consensus Decision Pathway for Periprocedural Management of Anticoagulation in Patients With Nonvalvular Atrial Fibrillation[11] recommends avoiding bridging for individuals at low thrombotic risk (CHA_2DS_2-VASc ≤4) with no history of thromboembolism and those at moderate thrombotic risk (CHA_2DS_2-VASc = 5-6) with increased bleed risk (history of major bleed or intracranial hemorrhage within the past 3 months, platelet abnormality, aspirin use, supratherapeutic international normalized ratio (INR), or prior bleed

[10]Douketis JD, et al. Perioperative bridging anticoagulation in patients with atrial fibrillation. *N Engl J Med.* 2015;373(9):823-833.

[11]Doherty JU, et al. 2017 ACC expert consensus decision pathway for periprocedural management of anticoagulation in patients with nonvalvular atrial fibrillation: a report of the American College of Cardiology Clinical Expert Consensus Document Task Force. *J Am Coll Cardiol.* 2017;69(7):871-898.

from previous anticoagulation bridging). In contrast, given the exclusions in BRIDGE, the guidelines recommend consideration of bridging anticoagulation in moderate-risk patients with remote history of thromboembolism and high-risk patients (CHA_2DS_2-VASc $\geq$ 7 or thromboembolism within the last 3 months) with high bleed risk. For high-risk patients without increased risk of bleed, bridging anticoagulation is strongly encouraged.

KEY LEARNING POINTS

1. Coronary revascularization is not recommended for patients with stable coronary artery disease prior to noncardiac surgery exclusively to decrease perioperative cardiac events.
2. Although perioperative β-blocker therapy can reduce risk of perioperative MI, initiation of beta-blocker therapy within 1 day of surgery or in patients considered low risk for perioperative cardiac complications can increase perioperative stroke and mortality.
3. The perioperative management of aspirin in patients undergoing noncardiac surgery remains controversial. Data suggest that perioperative aspirin therapy is associated with higher rates of major bleeding, with no significant reduction in rate of all-cause mortality and nonfatal MI. There may be cardiac morbidity and mortality benefit in patients with prior percutaneous coronary intervention.
4. Patients with atrial fibrillation who are on warfarin and considered low risk for stroke can avoid perioperative bridging anticoagulation, which increases bleeding risk without significantly reducing risk of thromboembolism.

ACUTE KIDNEY INJURY

Patrick Marcus, MD,
Eric M. LaMotte, MD

You are called by the ED to admit a 63-year-old man with a history of hypertension and type 2 diabetes mellitus to the ICU for sepsis from an unclear source. In the ED, blood cultures, lab work, chest radiograph, and urinalysis have been ordered. You note that the patient's Cr is 2.3 mg/dL at baseline. You consider which IV fluid to use for fluid resuscitation.

Among ICU patients, does the use of normal saline versus a buffered crystalloid solution impact the risk of acute kidney injury (AKI)?

For ICU patients, the choice of normal saline versus buffered crystalloid IV fluid does not appear to impact the incidence of AKI when administered in low volumes.

Given concerns that the supraphysiologic chloride concentration of normal saline may induce renal vasoconstriction and thus contribute to AKI, this question was studied in SPLIT,[1] a prospective, blinded, double cross-over cluster randomized controlled trial conducted among 2278 ICU patients at four academic centers in New Zealand. Patients were randomized to normal saline versus a proprietary buffered crystalloid solution (Plasma-Lyte) during their ICU stay. Individuals receiving or likely to receive renal replacement therapy (RRT) within 6 hours of admission were excluded. The primary outcome was the development of

---

[1]Young P, et al. Effect of a buffered crystalloid solution vs saline on acute kidney injury among patients in the intensive care unit: the SPLIT randomized clinical trial. *J Am Med Assoc.* 2015;314(16):1701-1710.

renal injury as defined by RIFLE (Risk, Injury, Failure, Loss, End-Stage Renal Disease) criteria: ≥2-fold increase in serum creatinine from baseline. Secondary outcomes included AKI by Kidney Disease: Improved Global Outcomes (KDIGO) criteria, RRT use, hospital mortality, and utilization measures (e.g., length-of-hospital, ICU stay).

The volume of fluid administered was comparable across groups (median 2000 mL for both groups; P = .63), with the majority of fluid administered in the first day of the ICU stay. No differences were observed in the development of AKI (9.6% in the buffered crystalloid group vs. 9.2% in the normal saline group, RR 1.04, 95% CI 0.80-1.36; P = .77), RRT use (3.3% in the buffered crystalloid group vs. 3.4%, in the normal saline group, RR 0.96, 95% CI 0.62-1.50; P = .91), or hospital mortality (7.6% in the buffered crystalloid group vs. 8.6%, in the normal saline group, RR 0.88, 95% CI, 0.67-1.17; P = .40). There were also no differences in ICU or hospital stays. Study caveats include large proportions of patients admitted to the ICU after cardiac surgery and confidence intervals too wide to definitively exclude meaningful clinical effects, which may not have been detected, given low volumes of administered fluids.

The association between type of fluid and renal dysfunction was further evaluated in the SMART trial,[2] a prospective cluster randomized trial of 15,000 ICU patients who were randomized to buffered crystalloid versus normal saline for initial resuscitation. The primary outcome was major adverse kidney events at 30 days (defined as the incidence of death, new RRT, or persistent elevation of creatinine over twice the baseline). Secondary outcomes included stage 2 or greater AKI (defined via KDIGO criteria).

The primary outcome occurred less frequently in patients receiving balanced crystalloid in the overall cohort (14.3% vs. 15.4%; P = .04), with differences driven by higher mortality among patients receiving normal saline, as well as in a prespecified subgroup of patients admitted with sepsis (33.8% vs. 38.9%; P = .01). Occurrence of stage 2 or greater AKI did not differ by type of fluid (10.7% vs. 11.5%; P = .09). As in SPLIT, the generalizability of findings from SMART is hindered by relatively low volume of administered fluids.

Nonetheless, consistent with the lack of clear impact of fluid type on AKI demonstrated by these studies, the 2016 Surviving Sepsis Campaign guidelines do not establish a preference between buffered crystalloid and normal saline during initial resuscitation.

---

[2]Semler MW, et al. Balanced crystalloids versus saline in critically ill adults. *N Engl J Med.* 2018;378(9)829-839.

While awaiting results from a work-up of potential sources of sepsis, you decide to treat the patient empirically with normal saline and broad-spectrum antibiotics.

Which broad-spectrum antibiotics pose the greatest risk of causing AKI?

Compared to other commonly used broad-spectrum antibiotic regimens, the combination of vancomycin and piperacillin/tazobactam is associated with the greatest risk of nephrotoxicity.

This question was addressed by a 2017 meta-analysis[3] that incorporated 15 published studies and 17 abstracts encompassing 24,799 patients who received one of the following regimens: vancomycin alone, piperacillin/tazobactam alone, vancomycin plus piperacillin/tazobactam, or vancomycin plus cefepime or a carbapenem. The primary outcome was AKI (defined by each individual study but most commonly based on AKIN, RIFLE, or KDIGO guidelines).

AKI was more likely with vancomycin plus piperacillin/tazobactam compared to vancomycin alone (OR 3.4, 95% CI 2.6-4.5; $P \le .01$), vancomycin plus cefepime or carbapenem (OR 2.7, 95% CI 1.8-3.9; $P \le .01$), and piperacillin-tazobactam alone (OR 2.7, 95% CI 2.0-3.7; $P \le .01$). The corresponding number needed to harm (NNH) for vancomycin plus piperacillin/tazobactam versus all other groups combined was 11.

These findings were corroborated by a 2018 prospective observational study[4] that evaluated the incidence of AKI among 242 adults at four US medical centers who received one of four regimens: ≥72 hours of vancomycin along with ≥48 hours of overlap with either (1) piperacillin/tazobactam, (2) meropenem, or (3) cefepime. Patients were excluded if they experienced AKI at any point prior to administration of antibiotics, or if their vancomycin trough or random levels were <10 mg/L, or baseline serum creatinine was >1.5 mg/dL. 37% carried a diagnosis of sepsis, with 15% of all patients having severe sepsis or septic shock. The primary outcome was AKI, defined as serum creatinine >1.5 times baseline within 7 days of antibiotic use.

---

[3]Luther M, et al. Vancomycin Plus Piperacillin-Tazobactam and acute kidney injury in adults: a systematic review and meta-analysis. *Crit Care Med.* 2018;46(1)12-20.

[4]Mullins B, et al. Comparison of the nephrotoxicity of vancomycin in combination with cefepime, meropenem, or piperacillin/tazobactam: a prospective, multicenter study. *Ann Pharmacother.* 2018:1-6.

AKI developed in 29.8% of patients receiving vancomycin and piperacillin/tazobactam compared to a combined 8.8% of patients receiving cefepime or meropenem ($P < .001$). Caveats include observational design and risk for misclassification bias. Together, both studies provide important information about the association between certain antibiotics and AKI that can be incorporated with other practices (e.g., use of local sensitivity patterns) to inform empiric antibiotic selection.

You initiate the patient on vancomycin and cefepime pending culture results. The patient's blood pressure remains normal without the need for vasopressors. However, given his elevated creatinine and high risk for further renal injury, the resident on your team asks you if low-dose dopamine may be appropriate to "protect his kidneys."

What is the role of dopamine infusions in nephroprotection among acutely ill patients?

There is no evidence to support the use of dopamine for nephroprotection in patients already showing evidence of sepsis and AKI.

The notion of nephroprotection—which stems from historical evidence that dopamine increases glomerular filtration rate (GFR) and renal blood flow in healthy subjects—was addressed in a multicenter, placebo-controlled trial[5] randomizing 328 ICU patients to continuous low-dose dopamine (2 mcg/kg/min) infusion versus placebo. Inclusion criteria included a combination of ≥2 systemic inflammatory response syndrome (SIRS) criteria and evidence of early renal dysfunction (oliguria for >4 hours, Cr elevated >150 μmol/L (1.7 mg/dL) in the absence of baseline renal dysfunction, or an acute rise in Cr of >80 μmol/L (0.9 mg/dL) over baseline). The primary outcome was peak serum Cr during the infusion, and secondary outcomes included ICU stay, hospital stay, and need for RRT.

There were no between-group differences with respect to the primary outcome (245 vs. 249 μmol/L; $P = .93$) or any of the secondary outcomes, including need for RRT (35 vs. 40 patients; $P = .55$) and ICU days (13 vs. 14 days; $P = .67$) or hospital stay (29 vs. 33 days; $P = .29$). Caveats include the fact that the degree of hypotension and need for additional vasopressors among participants were not well described.

[5]Bellomo R, et al. Low-dose dopamine in patients with early renal dysfunction: a placebo-controlled randomised trial. Lancet. 2000;356(9248):2139-2143.

Nonetheless, this study supported the class 1A KDIGO AKI practice guideline recommendation *against* the use of low-dose dopamine for preventing or treating AKI.[6]

The patient's sepsis physiology and renal function improve over the next 12 hours, and he appears clinically euvolemic on treatment with vancomycin, cefepime, and IV fluids. However, he develops acute abdominal pain, and you determine that the most appropriate test for evaluating this pain is an abdominal CT with IV contrast. You are concerned about potential contrast-induced nephropathy (CIN) and consider the role of fluid administration and N-acetylcysteine (NAC) in reducing his risk of developing CIN.

What is the role of fluid administration and NAC in preventing CIN in patients at high risk due to abnormal GFR?

The choice of IV fluid does not affect the risk of developing CIN in high-risk patients, and NAC administration prior to contrast does not reduce CIN risk. IV fluid administration appears to be more effective than oral hydration in reducing CIN.

Given the generally accepted notion that patients with abnormal GFR either from AKI or chronic kidney disease (CKD) are at higher risk for CIN, the PRESERVE trial[7] used a 2 × 2 factorial design to randomize 5177 patients with stage 3A (with diabetes), 3B, or 4 CKD to IV 1.26% sodium bicarbonate versus 0.9% sodium chloride, and either 5 days of oral NAC versus placebo prior to scheduled angiography. The primary outcome was a composite of death, increase in serum Cr by 50% at 90 days, or need for hemodialysis. CIN (defined as an increase in serum Cr by ≥0.5 mg/dL or 25% of baseline between 3 and 5 days after contrast exposure) was a secondary outcome.

The primary outcome did not differ based on choice of IV fluid (4.4% of patients receiving sodium bicarbonate group vs. 4.7% of patients receiving sodium chloride, OR 0.93, 95% CI 0.72-1.22; $P = .62$) or administration of NAC (4.6% vs. 4.5% among those who

---

[6]Kidney Disease Outcomes Quality Initiative. KDIGO clinical practice guidelines for acute kidney injury. *Kidney Int Suppl.* 2012;2(8).

[7]Weisbord SD, et al. Outcomes after angiography with sodium bicarbonate and acetylcysteine. *N Engl J Med.* 2018;378(7):603-614.

did and did not receive it, respectively, OR 1.02, 95% CI 0.78-1.33; $P = .88$). Among patients receiving either type of IV fluids, CIN did not differ between those receiving versus not receiving NAC. Importantly, patients in PRESERVE received relatively low doses of iso-osmolar or low-osmolar nonionic contrast agents.

Several studies have demonstrated efficacy of IV fluid administration over oral hydration in reducing CIN. One trial[8] randomized 53 patients with mean serum creatinine of 1.3 mg/dL to 12 hours of IV normal saline at 1 mL/kg/h versus 24 hours of unrestricted oral hydration prior to scheduled coronary angiography. CIN was defined as an increase in serum creatinine by ≥0.5 mg/dL within 48 hours of contrast exposure. Patients receiving IV fluids had significantly lower rates of CIN (4% vs. 35%, RR 0.11, 95% CI 0.015-0.79; $P = .005$). No patients required RRT.

KDIGO AKI guidelines give a 1A recommendation for IV hydration to prevent CIN and do not favor a specific type of IV fluid.

The patient receives IV normal saline prior to undergoing his abdominal CT with contrast, which demonstrates diverticulitis. He is transferred from the ICU to the acute care floor, antibiotics are transitioned to ciprofloxacin and metronidazole, and he is discharged home after further clinical improvement.

KEY LEARNING POINTS

1. For ICU patients, the choice of normal saline versus buffered crystalloid IV fluid does not appear to impact the incidence of AKI when administered in low volumes.
2. Compared to other commonly used broad-spectrum antibiotic regimens, the combination of vancomycin and piperacillin/tazobactam is associated with the greatest risk of nephrotoxicity.
3. There is no evidence to support the use of dopamine for nephroprotection in patients already showing evidence of sepsis and AKI.
4. The choice of IV fluid does not affect the risk of developing CIN in high-risk patients, and NAC administration prior to contrast does not reduce CIN risk. IV fluid administration appears to be more effective than oral hydration in reducing CIN.

---

[8]Trivedi HS, et al. A randomized prospective trial to assess the role of saline hydration on the development of contrast nephrotoxicity. *Nephron Clin Pract*. 2003;93:C29-C34.

OPIATES AND OPIATE USE DISORDER

Rachel Hensel, MD,
Zahir Kanjee, MD, MPH

You are admitting a 57-year-old opiate-naive woman with a history of obesity and obstructive sleep apnea (OSA) for pain control of a nonoperative fractured radius after a mechanical fall. Her pain is refractory to nonsteroidal anti-inflammatory drugs (NSAIDs) and acetaminophen. You start her on oral morphine with occasional IV breakthrough doses as needed. You worry about her risk of oversedation.

Which patient-related risk factors are most associated with opiate-induced oversedation in the hospital?

Several comorbidities—especially congestive heart failure, acute kidney injury, and OSA—and concurrent central nervous system (CNS)-depressant medication are most associated with oversedation from opiates in the hospital.

A study conducted at a large US academic medical center in 2011 used institutional data on all 32 respiratory emergencies among postoperative patients referred to risk management from August 2000 to July 2007 to identify risk factors for opiate-related respiratory events.[1] Events were eligible for inclusion as respiratory emergencies if the patient received opiates and subsequently suffered unresponsiveness with hypoxia/apnea requiring administration of naloxone or a cardiac arrest deemed to be primarily respiratory in etiology.

[1] Ramachandran SK, et al. Life-threatening critical respiratory events: a retrospective study of postoperative patients found unresponsive during analgesic therapy. *J Clin Anesth.* 2011;23(3):207-213.

TABLE 26.1

Comorbidity and OR for Opioid-Related Respiratory Event

Comorbidity	Unadjusted OR (95% CI)
Congestive heart failure	34.9 (13.6-90.1)
Postoperative acute kidney injury	18.6 (5.8-59.5)
OSA	16.9 (8.3-34.5)
Dysrhythmia	5.3 (2.2-12.5)
Diabetes mellitus	4.7 (1.8-12.1)
Coronary artery disease	3.1 (1.3-7.0)
Hypertension	1.9 (1.1-3.9)

OSA, obstructive sleep apnea.

Data adapted from Ramachandran SK, et al. Life-threatening critical respiratory events: a retrospective study of postoperative patients found unresponsive during analgesic therapy. *J Clin Anesth.* 2011;23(3):207-213.

The charts for all identified respiratory emergencies during the study period were reviewed to assess patient demographics, comorbidities, timing in relation to anesthesia cessation, and details on opiate administration. Characteristics for these 32 patients were compared to those of control patients admitted to the hospital after receiving postanesthesia care without experiencing a respiratory emergency during the study period.

The majority of respiratory emergencies (81.3%) occurred within the first 24 hours after anesthesia, and 12.5% were fatal. Compared to control patients, those with opiate-related respiratory events were more likely to have a number of comorbidities (Table 26.1). This analysis was limited by study design (retrospective, single center, based on risk management identification of events), small sample size of primarily surgical patients, and the lack of multivariable adjustment for confounders.

A 2014 retrospective case-control study evaluated risk factors for the use of rescue naloxone in 65 patients at a single medium-sized US community teaching hospital.[2] Adult patients ≥18 years old were included as cases if they were administered ≥1 dose of naloxone between October 2011 and September 2012, and their electronic chart review indicated

---

[2]Pawasauskas J, et al. Predictors of naloxone use for respiratory depression and oversedation in hospitalized adults. *Am J Health Syst Pharm.* 2014;71(9):746-750.

TABLE 26.2

Risk Factors for Naloxone Administration

Risk Factor	OR (95% CI)
Renal disease	6.034 (2.565-14.195)
Cardiac disease	5.829 (2.687-12.642)
Concurrent CNS depressant	4.750 (1.949-11.578)
Smoking history	4.421 (2.114-9.245)
Pulmonary disease	3.600 (1.742-7.441)
Opiate naive	0.317 (0.150-0.667)

CNS, central nervous system.

Reprinted from Pawasauskas J, et al. Predictors of naloxone use for respiratory depression and oversedation in hospitalized adults. *Am J Health Syst Pharm.* 2014;71(9):746-750, with permission from Oxford University Press.

oversedation, respiratory depression, or improvement after naloxone. Patients were excluded as cases if their naloxone administration occurred within 24 hours of admission; in an ED, operating room, or postanesthesia unit; or was not preceded by an opiate in the prior 24 hours. The 65 case patients were matched with controls who had similar (80%-120%) 24-hour equivalent opiate administration. Potential risk factors analyzed by logistic regression included demographic characteristics, nursing unit, body mass index (BMI), smoking history, opiate naivete (assessed by preadmission medication reconciliation), concurrent CNS depressant use, or presence of pulmonary, renal, cardiac, or hepatic disease.

Several factors were found to be associated with naloxone administration (Table 26.2). Study caveats include its retrospective case-control and single-centered design, small sample size, and the inability to definitively assess opiate use prior to admission beyond preadmission medication reconciliation, which likely missed illicit and nonprescription opiate use.

The Society of Hospital Medicine (SHM) guidelines[3] recommend "extra caution" with opiates in the setting of a number of the conditions listed above and avoiding coprescription with other CNS-depressant medications when possible.

---

[3]Herzig SJ, et al. Improving the safety of opioid use for acute noncancer pain in hospitalized adults: a consensus statement from the Society of Hospital Medicine. *J Hosp Med.* 2018;13(4):263-271.

You order continuous pulse oximetry and work with nursing staff to monitor the patient closely for oversedation given her OSA. Over the course of 2 days, she is able to wean down her opiate usage to only occasional low-dose oral morphine as needed prior to discharge. Given the persistence of her pain, she would like to be discharged with a short course of opiates at home but also expresses concern about her risk for chronic opiate use.

Does an opiate prescription on discharge increase the risk that an opiate-naive patient will use this class of medications chronically?

Receiving opiates on discharge can increase the likelihood of chronic use among opiate-naive patients.

This question was assessed by a 2016 retrospective cohort study conducted among 6689 patients ≥15 years of age discharged from a large US academic safety net hospital-based system.[4] Each patient was assigned an index admission and discharge based on the first hospitalization during the 12-month study period. Exclusion criteria included prior opiate use (filling of an opiate prescription at an affiliated pharmacy within the preceding 12 months), death during the index admission, hemodialysis, or <2 visits in the healthcare system. The primary exposure was opiate receipt (filling of a prescription at an affiliated pharmacy <72 hours from index discharge). The primary outcome was chronic use (either >10 filled opiate prescriptions or receipt of ≥120 days' supply and >90 days duration) during the following year. Secondary outcomes included the number of additional opiate dispensations within 12 months following index discharge. Covariates included demographics (including insurance status); diagnosis of chronic pain, acute pain, cancer, and psychiatric disease (including substance use); number of later readmissions during the year; and Charlson Comorbidity Index.

A large proportion (25%) of patients received an opiate on discharge. In multivariable analysis, opiate receipt was associated with chronic use (OR 4.90, 95% CI 3.22-7.45; no *P*-value reported). Other factors associated with increased odds of chronic use included diagnosis of chronic pain (OR 2.24, 95% CI 1.16-4.30; no *P*-value reported), increasing Charlson Comorbidity Index (OR 1.22, 95% CI 1.13-1.33; no *P*-value reported), and number of readmissions during that year (OR 2.02, 95%

[4]Calcaterra SL, et al. Opioid prescribing at hospital discharge contributes to chronic opioid use. *J Gen Intern Med.* 2016;31(5):478-485.

CI 1.80-2.27; no *P*-value reported). Patients with Medicare insurance (OR 0.50, 95% CI 0.28-0.92; no *P*-value reported) and cancer diagnosis (OR 0.30, 95% CI 0.12-0.76; no *P*-value reported) had reduced odds of chronic use. Study caveats include retrospective single-centered design and reliance on data from pharmacies affiliated with one system.

Consistent with concerns about issues associated with chronic opiate use, SHM guidelines[5] advise discussing risks of opiates such as physical dependence and addiction when deciding whether to prescribe these medications.

> You discuss the risks and benefits of a short course of opiate therapy with the patient. You include the primary care physician (PCP) in the process of shared decision-making and ultimately prescribe her a very short course on discharge. You would like to order the opiate in a way that is least likely to lead to long-term use or harm.

Which prescription-related factors are associated with long-term use and unintentional overdose in the opiate-naive population?

Among opiate-naive patients, initial prescriptions with higher daily doses and greater days' supply are associated with long-term opiate use, while long-acting formulations are associated with unintentional overdose.

Factors related to long-term opiate use were evaluated in a 2018 retrospective observational study conducted within the Veterans Health Administration (VA) system.[6] Patients were included if they had an outpatient prescription for a noninjectable opiate during 2011 and had not received opiates in the year prior. Exclusion criteria included metastatic cancer, palliative care, and opiate dependence treatment. The primary outcome was long-term opiate use, "defined as an episode of continuous opiate supply for >90 days and beginning within 30 days of the initial prescription." Covariates included index prescription details (such as dose in morphine mg equivalents per day and days' supply), patient demographics, diagnosis, substance use disorder, mental health disorder, chronic pain, concurrent benzodiazepine use, and urban or rural residence.

---

[5]Herzig SJ, et al. Improving the safety of opioid use for acute noncancer pain in hospitalized adults: a consensus statement from the Society of Hospital Medicine. *J Hosp Med.* 2018;13(4):263-271.

[6]Mosher HJ, et al. Predictors of long-term opioid use after opioid initiation at discharge from medical and surgical hospitalizations. *J Hosp Med.* 2018;13(4):243-248.

In multivariable analysis, factors associated with long-term use included a higher dose and longer duration on the index script (Table 26.3) as well as chronic pain diagnosis (OR 1.18, 95% CI 1.04-1.21; no *P*-value reported) and muscle relaxant use either concurrent to the index prescription (OR 1.69, 95% CI 1.52-1.89; no *P*-value reported) or within the preceding year (OR 1.17, 95% CI 1.01-1.35; no *P*-value reported). Study limitations included decreased generalizability due to the use of only VA patients and VA pharmacy records.

Another retrospective study in the VA system evaluated the association between the duration of action of the opiate prescribed and the risk of unintentional overdose.[7] Patients were included if they possessed a diagnosis of chronic noncancer pain and filled ≥ 1 opiate prescription during the study period (2000-2009) within the VA system. For each eligible patient, the first opiate prescription filled during the study period without another opiate prescription in the preceding 6 months was defined as the index prescription. Exclusion criteria included hospice status in the year prior to

TABLE 26.3

Risk Factors on Index Prescription for Subsequent Chronic Opiate Use

Covariate on Index Prescription	OR (95% CI)
Morphine equivalents (mg/day)	
≤15	Referent
15.01-30	1.11 (1.02-1.21)
30.01-45	1.18 (1.05-1.33)
>45	1.70 (1.49-1.94)
Supply (days)	
≤7	Referent
8-14	1.24 (1.12-1.37)
15-29	1.56 (1.39-1.76)
≥30	2.59 (2.35-2.86)

Adapted from Mosher HJ, et al. Predictors of long-term opioid use after opioid initiation at discharge from medical and surgical hospitalizations. *J Hosp Med.* 2018;13(4):243-248.

---

[7]Miller M, et al. Prescription opioid duration of action and the risk of unintentional overdose among patients receiving opioid therapy. *JAMA Intern Med.* 2015;175(4):608-615.

the index prescription. Opiates were classified as long-acting (excluding liquid methadone because it is the primary agent used in the VA system for maintenance therapy) or short-acting. The primary outcome was unintentional overdose (excluding events that were caused by external injury, self-infliction, or assault). Other covariates included demographics, disability, medical and psychiatric disorders, mental health and substance disorder treatment, ED visits, hospitalizations, and nonopiate pain medications. Patients were censored at earliest occurrence of the following events: overdose, change of opiate agent, death, discontinuation of opiate treatment, hospice entry, ineligibility for VA benefits, or study end. Doses were converted to oral morphine equivalents. To minimize bias, a propensity score was used for inverse probability weighting.

After adjustment, use of long-acting opiates was associated with a higher risk of unintentional overdose (HR 2.33, 95% CI 1.26-4.32; no *P*-value reported). This risk of overdose was higher during the first 14 days of therapy (HR 5.25, 95% CI 1.88-14.72; no *P*-value reported) compared to days 15 to 60 (HR 2.30, 95% CI 0.67-7.90; no *P*-value reported) and >60 days (HR 1.50, 95% CI 0.68-3.33; no *P*-value reported). Study caveats include retrospective design, use of administrative data, and limitation to only VA patients.

SHM recommends prescribing the minimum necessary quantity of immediate-release (rather than long-acting) opiates for acute pain on hospital discharge.[8]

> You send the patient home with a short duration of low-dose immediate-release opiates as needed with advice to follow-up with her PCP. When you check her records several months later, you see she has not needed any further opiate prescriptions.
>
> Also on your service is a 38-year-old man with a history of opiate use disorder (OUD) with active injection drug use who presents after an accidental overdose and aspiration pneumonia. He improves rapidly with medical management. He is interested in stopping his use of illicit drugs. You consider initiation of medication-assisted therapy (MAT) such as buprenorphine, methadone maintenance therapy (MMT), and naltrexone, but he is hesitant and wants to know whether this will really help him.

---

[8]Herzig SJ, et al. Improving the safety of opioid use for acute noncancer pain in hospitalized adults: a consensus statement from the Society of Hospital Medicine. *J Hosp Med.* 2018;13(4):263-271.

What are the benefits of MAT for OUD patients who survive opiate overdose?

MAT, in particular buprenorphine and MMT, is associated with reductions in mortality among OUD patients who survive overdose.

A large retrospective cohort study using statewide registries and databases evaluated the association between MAT (MMT, buprenorphine, or naltrexone) and mortality among 17,568 survivors of opiate overdose in Massachusetts.[9] Adult patients (≥18 years old) were included if they had a nonfatal opiate overdose (using validated medical claims and ambulance data) during the study period, with the first episode defined as the index event. Patients were excluded if they had cancer (by claims or a statewide registry) or died within 30 days of the index event. The exposure of interest was receipt of MAT (from medical and pharmacy claims, state addiction treatment databases, and the state prescription monitoring program). Covariates included demographics, opiate and benzodiazepine receipt, anxiety or depression, and treatment in inpatient and residential detoxification facilities. The primary outcomes were all-cause and opiate-related (based on medical examiner or Department of Public Health assessment) mortality during the subsequent year.

In multivariable analysis, MMT and buprenorphine were each associated with reductions in all-cause and opiate-related mortality compared

TABLE 26.4

All-Cause Mortality and Opioid-Related Mortality for MAT Modalities Compared to No MAT

	All-Cause Mortality, HR (95% CI)	Opiate-Related Mortality, HR (95% CI)
No MAT	Referent	Referent
MMT	0.47 (0.32-0.71)	0.41 (0.24-0.70)
Buprenorphine	0.63 (0.46-0.87)	0.62 (0.41-0.92)
Naltrexone	1.44 (0.84-2.46)	1.43 (0.73-2.79)

MMT, methadone maintenance therapy.

Data from Larochelle MR, et al. Medication for opioid use disorder after nonfatal opioid overdose and association with mortality. *Ann Int Med.* 2018; 169(3):137-145.

---

[9]Larochelle MR, et al. Medication for opioid use disorder after nonfatal opioid overdose and association with mortality. *Ann Int Med.* 2018;169(3):137-145.

to no MAT (Table 26.4). Study caveats include the observational design, use of administrative data, and limitation to one state.

The Centers for Disease Control and Prevention (CDC) recommends the use of buprenorphine or MMT for treatment of OUD.[10]

KEY LEARNING POINTS

1. Several comorbidities—especially congestive heart failure, acute kidney injury, and OSA—and concurrent CNS-depressant medication are most associated with oversedation from opiates in the hospital.
2. Receiving opiates on discharge can increase the likelihood of chronic use among opiate-naive patients.
3. Among opiate-naive patients, initial prescriptions with higher daily doses and greater days' supply are associated with long-term opiate use, while long-acting formulations are associated with unintentional overdose.
4. MAT, particularly buprenorphine and MMT, is associated with reduced mortality in OUD patients who survive overdose.

---

[10]Dowell D, et al. CDC guideline for prescribing opioids for chronic pain–United States, 2016. *J Am Med Assoc.* 2016;315(15):1624-1645.

HIP FRACTURE

Neal Biddick, MD,
Staci Saunders, MD,
Zahir Kanjee, MD, MPH

A 79-year-old woman with hypertension, diabetes, and chronic heart failure presents after a mechanical fall. She is admitted to an orthopedics-hospitalist comanagement service for operative repair of a hip fracture. You find her to be at acceptable risk and medically optimized for surgery. You consider whether the patient should undergo the operation within 24 hours of presentation or if she would have a similar outcome if she were to wait until later.

Is there a benefit to early (<24 hours) compared to late (>24 hours) surgery after hip fracture?

Complications and mortality are more common when patients wait >24 hours for surgery.

This question was evaluated by a 2017 analysis of administrative data for 42,230 patients undergoing hip fracture surgery performed by 522 orthopedic surgeons in Ontario, Canada.[1] Patients with previous hip fracture, lacking data on hospital arrival time, <45 years old, or receiving surgery by nonorthopedic surgeons were excluded. The primary exposure was time from initial presentation to any ED until surgery (in hours). Covariates included characteristics of patients (demographics, comorbidity [based on previously validated models]), orthopedic-specific conditions (osteomyelitis, bone cancer, other fracture, recent hip arthroplasty, and trauma), procedure (type, duration, and time of day/week), operating

---

[1]Pincus D, et al. Association between wait time and 30-day mortality in adults undergoing hip fracture surgery. *J Am Med Assoc.* 2017;318(20):1994-2003.

surgeons (seniority, volume), and hospital (surgical volume, size, and academic or community status). The primary outcome was 30-day mortality from time of admission. Secondary outcomes included 90-day and 1-year mortality as well as medical complications (including myocardial infarction, venous thromboembolism, and pneumonia).

After controlling for covariates, 30-day mortality was first analyzed using time as a continuous variable. A graphic depiction of this analysis permitted the selection of an inflection point in the primary exposure at which to dichotomize patients into early versus late surgery groups. A logistic regression with propensity-score matching was subsequently performed. Authors conducted multiple sensitivity analyses including one limited to patients without comorbidity, another among those >65 years of age who had received blood thinners within a year prior to surgery, and a *post hoc* analysis limited to patients undergoing surgery within 36 hours.

The mean time to surgery was 38.8 hours. An inflection point was notable at 24 hours (Figure 27.1), so this time point was chosen as the demarcation between the early and late surgery groups in further analyses. The primary outcome was lower in the early surgery group (5.8% vs. 6.5%, absolute risk reduction 0.79%, 95% CI 0.23%-1.35%; $P = .006$). The early surgery group also had reductions in 90-day (absolute risk reduction 1.35%, 95% CI 0.61%-2.10%; $P < .001$) and 1-year (absolute risk reduction 2.31%, 95% CI 1.47%-3.25%; $P < .001$) mortality, along with numerous outcomes at 30 days such as pulmonary embolism (absolute risk reduction 0.51%, 95% CI 0.28%-0.74%; $P < .001$), pneumonia (absolute risk reduction 0.95%, 95% CI 0.48-1.43; $P < .001$), and myocardial infarction (absolute risk reduction 0.39, 95% CI 0.15%-0.62%; $P = .001$). These results were robust to sensitivity analyses limited to patients without comorbidity, who underwent surgery within 36 hours, and >65 years of age who received blood thinner prescriptions in the previous year. Caveats include the retrospective design and use of administrative data.

National Institute for Health and Care Excellence (NICE) guidelines[2] recommend surgery on the same day or 1 day following admission.

> The patient undergoes an uncomplicated hemiarthroplasty the following morning, within 24 hours of arrival. After this traumatic experience, she is very afraid of breaking her other hip. Her renal function and levels of Ca and vitamin D are within normal limits. Some of her friends with osteoporosis are taking a bisphosphonate, and she asks if that would help her.

---

[2]National Institute for Health and Care Excellence. *Hip fracture: Management.* London: NICE; 2017. Available at: https://www.nice.org.uk/guidance/cg124. Accessed December 17, 2018.

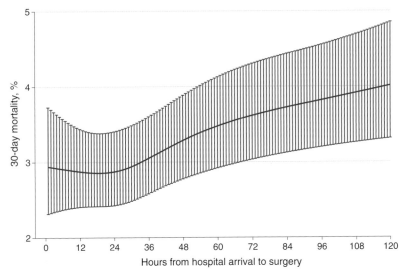

Figure 27.1 The relationship between hours from hospital arrival to surgery and 30-day mortality, adjusted for multiple covariates. (Reprinted from Pincus D, et al. Association between wait time and 30-day mortality in adults undergoing hip fracture surgery. *J Am Med Assoc.* 2017;318(20):1994-2003, with permission.)

Do intravenous bisphosphonates prevent adverse outcomes after an osteoporotic hip fracture?

Intravenous zoledronic acid prevents recurrent fractures and decreases mortality in patients with osteoporotic hip fractures.

HORIZON-RFT[3] was a multinational, randomized, double-blind, placebo-controlled trial of zoledronic acid, a once-yearly intravenous bisphosphonate, among 2127 patients with recent hip fracture. Previously ambulatory patients ≥50 years of age were included within 90 days from surgical hip fracture repair after low-intensity trauma (such as a fall from standing) if they refused or could not tolerate an oral bisphosphonate. Exclusion criteria included CrCl <30 mL/min, corrected Ca <8.0 mg/dL or >11.0 mg/dL, active cancer, or non-osteoporotic metabolic bone disease. Patients received zoledronic acid 5 mg IV annually or placebo within 90 days of surgical repair and were followed for up to 5 years. Initially, vitamin D_2 or D_3 loading doses 2 weeks prior to the study drug were reserved for those whose 25-hydroxyvitamin D was either ≤15 ng/mL

---

[3]Lyles KW, et al. Zoledronic acid and clinical fractures and mortality after hip fracture. *N Engl J Med.* 2007; 357(18):1799-1809.

or not available, but after the authors noted very high prevalence of vitamin D deficiency, the protocol was changed and all subsequent patients received loading doses routinely. All patients received routine oral daily supplementation of Ca and vitamin D. Patients underwent annual dual-energy x-ray absorptiometry scans.

The initial primary outcome was time to first fracture, but due to a low event rate, this plan was altered slightly during the course of the study. The subsequent primary outcome was new clinical fracture (outside of facial/digital fractures or those in abnormal, such as metastatic, bone). Secondary outcomes included rates of vertebral and non-vertebral fractures, changes in bone mineral density (BMD), delayed healing of the index fracture, osteonecrosis of the jaw, other adverse events, and mortality.

The trial was stopped early for efficacy. The zoledronic acid group had fewer clinical fractures (8.6% vs. 13.9%, HR 0.65, 95% CI 0.50-0.84; P = .001), with reductions in both non-vertebral (7.6% vs. 10.7%, HR 0.73, 95% CI 0.55-0.98; P = .03) and vertebral (1.7% vs. 3.8%, HR 0.54, 95% CI 0.32-0.92; P = .02) fractures. BMD showed improvements in the zoledronic acid group as compared to the placebo group at 12, 24, and 36 months at both the femoral neck and the total hip areas (P < .001 for each comparison). Mortality was lower in the zoledronic acid group (9.6% vs. 13.3%, HR 0.72, 95% CI 0.56-0.93; P = .01). There were no between-group differences in rate of renal events, osteonecrosis of the jaw, or delayed healing of the index hip fracture. Hypocalcemia was potentially more frequent in the zoledronic acid group (0.3% vs. 0%; P-value not reported).

Study caveats include the exclusion of patients amenable to/tolerant of oral bisphosphonates (potentially limiting generalizability), the vitamin D repletion regimen potentially limiting the rate of hypocalcemia, and the midtrial change in the primary outcome.

HORIZON-RFT is frequently extrapolated to oral bisphosphonates. American Association of Clinical Endocrinologists (AACE)/American College of Endocrinology (ACE) postmenopausal osteoporosis guidelines[4] strongly recommend pharmacologic treatment for osteopenic patients with spine or hip fragility fracture (grade A, level of evidence 1). Zoledronic acid is a key option, especially for patients at highest risk for subsequent fracture and those unable to tolerate oral bisphosphonates (grade A, level of evidence 1).

---

[4]Camacho PM, et al. American Association of Clinical Endocrinologists and American College of Endocrinology clinical practice guidelines for the diagnosis and treatment of postmenopausal osteoporosis–2016. *Endocrine Practice*. 2016;22(4):1-42.

You discuss the plan to initiate bisphosphonates with the orthopedic surgeon who performed the patient's surgery. She agrees that bisphosphonates are indicated, but raises the concern of poor fracture healing due to the mechanism of action of this medication class, and suggests waiting a few months before such treatment.

Is initiating bisphosphonate soon after surgery for osteoporotic hip fracture associated with reductions in fracture healing?

No, bisphosphonate therapy as early as 1 to 2 weeks postoperatively does not inhibit fracture healing.

A *post hoc* secondary analysis[5] of 2111 patients in HORIZON-RFT who received ≥1 dose of zoledronic acid assessed this question. The primary exposure was the timing of zoledronic acid infusion relative to fracture repair (<2, 2-4, 4-6, and >6 weeks). The primary outcome was delayed healing of the index fracture, as defined by the combination of radiographic findings and symptoms >6 weeks after surgery. The occurrence of this outcome was assessed via a blinded multidisciplinary panel that reviewed the patient's pre- and postoperative imaging and chart for definitive evidence of the primary outcome, with the panel triggered in one of two ways. First, patients underwent multiple in-person and telephone follow-up visits where they were evaluated for symptoms suggestive of the primary outcome. Second, a regulatory database and a World Health Organization (WHO) registry were searched for evidence of delayed healing in study patients. Multivariable logistic regression included covariates associated with the risk for poor healing (demographics, body mass index (BMI), fracture type, rheumatoid arthritis, diabetes, and NSAID use). Timing of zoledronic acid was not associated with delayed healing (OR 1.20, 95% CI 0.74-1.95; $P = .44$). Study caveats include *post hoc* nature, which increased the possibility of incident delayed healing cases not being ascertained by the study's methods.

A subsequent multicenter study[6] randomized 90 patients with intertrochanteric fracture to weekly risedronate starting either 1 week, 1 month, or

[5]Colon-Emeric C, et al. Association between timing of zoledronic acid infusion and hip fracture healing. *Osteoporos Int.* 2011;22(8):2329-2236.

[6]Kim TY, et al. Does early administration of bisphosphonate affect fracture healing in patients with intertrochanteric fractures? *J Bone Joint Surg Br.* 2012;94(7):956-960.

3 months postoperatively. Patients were included if they were ambulatory preoperatively, had BMD findings of osteoporosis, and had not received a bisphosphonate within the previous 2 years. Patients were excluded if they had chronic kidney disease. All patients received screw fixation or an intramedullary nail, Ca and vitamin D supplementation, and regular postoperative follow-up. The primary outcome was time to radiographic fracture healing as assessed by two study surgeons. Secondary outcomes included functional status (by Koval classification) at 1 year and revision surgery.

There were no differences in time to radiographic fracture healing (10.7 vs. 12.9 vs. 12.3 weeks in the 1 week, 1 month, and 3 month groups, respectively; $P = .420$) nor in functional status ($P = .948$) or rates of revision surgery ($P = .550$). Study caveats include small sample size and limited applicability to non-intertrochanteric fractures or those managed with alternate procedures.

You replete her low levels of vitamin D, and start her on a daily Ca and vitamin D supplement. You and the orthopedic surgeon both advise her primary care physician (PCP) to start a bisphosphonate a few weeks after discharge.

A few months later, the patient re-presents with subacute hip pain at the site of her surgery. She has had no systemic symptoms or trauma, and the joint is without erythema, warmth, or drainage. Radiographs are unremarkable without evidence of poor healing or obvious surgical complication. She is admitted to your service for pain control.

You consult orthopedic surgery, and together, you consider the possibility that the patient has a chronic (>6 weeks from surgery) periprosthetic joint infection (PJI). An arthrocentesis is performed. In the absence of clear signs of PJI (such as purulence, a draining sinus tract, or rapidly growing cultures), you wonder how to interpret blood and synovial fluid results.

In the absence of clear signs of PJI, which serum or synovial fluid findings are most helpful for diagnosing chronic hip PJI?

Serum erythrocyte sedimentation rate (ESR) and CRP as well as synovial WBC count and polymorphonuclear percentage (PMN%) are useful for the diagnosis of PJI, with combinations of tests being particularly helpful. Synovial fluid WBC count values that raise suspicion for PJI are lower than those for native joint infection.

A 2008 single-centered prospective cohort study evaluated diagnostic utility of several serum and synovial tests for PJI in 220 consecutive patients undergoing revision after prosthetic hip implantation at a single academic orthopedic center.[7] Patients were excluded if they received preoperative antibiotics, had a draining sinus tract, or a preexisting diagnosis of inflammatory arthritis. All patients had routine serum ESR and CRP testing, hip aspiration for WBC count and differential, as well as intraoperative deep joint culture, frozen-section, and histopathological evaluation. A receiver operating characteristic curve was created to assess optimal an optimal cut-point for synovial WBC count and % PMN. PJI was considered present if two of the following three criteria were met: positive intraoperative culture, gross purulence, or histopathologic evidence of infection.

Mean interval between prosthetic hip implantation and revision surgery was 7.2 years, and PJI was diagnosed in 27.4%. Results are displayed in Table 27.1. Elevated ESR and CRP were each very sensitive for PJI. Among all patients, the optimal cut-point for synovial WBC count and PMN% was 4200 cells/mL and 80%, respectively. Among those with

TABLE 27.1

Diagnostic Performance of Tests for PJI

Test	Sensitivity (95% CI)	Specificity (95% CI)
ESR >30 mm/h	97% (93%-100%)	39% (31%-47%)
CRP >10 mg/dL	94% (87%-100%)	71% (64%-79%)
Synovial fluid WBC count >4200 cells/mL	84% (74%-94%)	93% (88%-98%)
Synovial fluid WBC count >3000 cells/mL in those with elevated ESR and CRP	90% (82%-98%)	91% (85%-97%)
Synovial fluid PMN% >80%	84% (74%-93%)	82% (76%-89%)

PJI, periprosthetic joint infection.

Data from Schinsky MF, et al. Perioperative testing for joint infection in patients undergoing revision total hip arthroplasty. *J Bone Joint Surg.* 2008;90(9):1869-1875.

---

[7]Schinsky MF, et al. Perioperative testing for joint infection in patients undergoing revision total hip arthroplasty. *J Bone Joint Surg.* 2008;90(9):1869-1875.

both elevated ESR and CRP, the optimal synovial WBC count cut-point was 3000 cells/mL (sensitivity 90%, specificity 91%). These WBC cut-points are notably much lower for PJI than those traditionally used for native hip infection.

Caveats to this study include single-centered design and prolonged mean duration between prosthetic hip implantation and revision surgery (subsequent studies have divided PJI into acute and chronic phases, using different diagnostic thresholds of the same tests above for each) and potential selection bias from inclusion of only patients proceeding to surgery.

The 2014 Infectious Diseases Society of America (IDSA) guidelines recommend checking ESR and CRP for all cases of suspected PJI (strength of recommendation A, level of evidence III) and arthrocentesis (unless surgery is planned or if it would not change management) with analysis of synovial fluid cell count and differential (strength of recommendation A, level of evidence III).[8]

Based on serum (ESR 65 mm/h, CRP 25 mg/dL) and synovial findings (WBC 4900 cells/mL, 85% PMN), suspicion for PJI is high. The patient proceeds to surgery, where histopathology confirms infection. Together with the patient, the orthopedic surgeon, and an infectious disease consultant, you devise a plan of care.

KEY LEARNING POINTS

1. Complications and mortality are more common when patients wait >24 hours for hip fracture surgery.
2. Intravenous zoledronic acid prevents recurrent fractures and decreases mortality in patients with osteoporotic hip fractures.
3. Bisphosphonate therapy as early as 1 to 2 weeks after hip fracture does not inhibit fracture healing.
4. In the absence of clear findings, serum (ESR and CRP) and synovial (WBC count, PMN%) tests are useful for the diagnosis of PJI, with combinations of tests being particularly helpful. Synovial fluid WBC count values that raise suspicion for PJI are lower than those for native joint infection.

---

[8]Osmon DR, et al. Diagnosis and management of prosthetic joint infection: Clinical practice guidelines by the Infectious Diseases Society of America. *Clin Infect Dis.* 2013;56(1):e1-e25.

FRAILTY IN HOSPITALIZED PATIENTS

Leah Marcotte, MD,
Joshua M. Liao, MD, MSc

You are consulted by vascular surgery on the care of an 88-year-old woman admitted to their service for threatened limb with plans to undergo lower extremity bypass procedure. She lives in an assisted living facility, uses a walker for ambulation, and has heart failure with preserved ejection fraction. The admitting resident physician requested a medicine consultation for perioperative risk evaluation and noted she was concerned because the patient appeared "frail."

Which instruments may be used to assess frailty in hospitalized patients?

Numerous instruments have been developed to evaluate frailty in hospitalized patients, including several versions of the Risk Analysis Index (RAI) among surgical patients and Canadian Study of Health and Aging Clinical Frailty Scale (CSHA-CFS) among medical patients.

Two versions of the RAI, the clinical (RAI-C) and administrative (RAI-A), were developed and validated in a 2017 study to evaluate frailty among surgical patients.[1] Variables included in the RAI-C were selected from the Minimum Data Set Mortality Risk Index-Revised using stepwise logistic regression to identify those that most reliably predicted 6-month mortality. The RAI-A was comprised of variables in the Veterans Affairs and American College of Surgeons National Surgical Quality Improvement Project (VASQIP and ACS-NSQIP) that most closely corresponded to variables in the RAI-C.

---

[1]Hall DE, et al. Development and initial validation of the risk analysis index for measuring frailty in surgical populations. *JAMA Surg.* 2017;152(2):175-182.

The RAI-C, scored on a scale of 0 to 81, was validated using data from 6856 patients at outpatient Veterans Health Administration surgery clinics in Nebraska and Western Iowa between July 2011 and September 2015. Information for 2785 patients with available VASQIP and ACS-NSQIP data was used to validate the RAI-A. Primary outcomes were 30-day, 180-day, and 365-day mortality. Secondary outcomes included postoperative complications. Instrument performance was assessed using C statistics, sensitivity, and specificity.

Among the 2785 patients with data available to calculate both the RAI-C and RAI-A, the C statistics for predicting mortality ranged from 0.744 to 0.824 for the RAI-C and from 0.797 to 0.901 with the RAI-A. Using a cutoff of 21 points utilized in prior studies, the RAI-C had a sensitivity of 50% and specificity of 82%, compared to a sensitivity of 25% and specificity of 97% for the RAI-A. Study caveats included potential bias from incomplete morbidity and mortality data.

The CSHA-CFS was developed and validated as part of a 5-year prospective cohort study conducted among 2305 community dwelling adults ≥65 years of age without dementia.[2] CSHA-CFS is a 7-point scale of increasing frailty that was derived from the authors' earlier theoretical model of fitness and frailty (Table 28.1). Study physicians examined and assigned a CSHA-CFS score for each study participant. Primary outcomes were death and need for institutional care.

Overall, higher CSHA-CFS scores were associated with the primary outcomes (HR 1.30 for death, 95% CI 1.27-1.33; HR 1.46 for institutional care, 95% CI 1.39-1.53; P-value not reported). Incremental 1-category change along the CSHA-CFS scale was associated with mortality (21%, 95% CI 13%-31%; P-value not reported) and need for institutional care (24%, 95% CI 9%-41%; P-value not reported). Study caveats include a disproportionately large number of individuals in the study cohort with cognitive impairment and living in institutional facilities.

A 2013 consensus statement[3] from six international professional societies recommend screening for frailty using a validated tool (without preference among available tools) in all adults >70 years of age.

> You complete your consultative evaluation and deem the patient to be frail based on a RAI-C score of 21. The vascular surgeon asks you how this might affect the decision to proceed with surgery.

[2]Rockwood K, et al. A global clinical measure of fitness and frailty in elderly people. *Can Med Assoc J.* 2005;173(5):489-495.

[3]Morley JE, et al. Frailty consensus: a call to action. *J Am Med Dir Assoc.* 2013;14(6):392-397.

TABLE 28.1

Canadian Study of Health and Aging Clinical Frailty Scale (CSHA-CFS)

Category	Category Description
1	Very fit (energetic, motivated, exercise regularly)
2	Well (no active disease, less fit than category 1)
3	Well, with treated comorbid disease
4	Apparently vulnerable (not frankly dependent, disease symptoms, slowed up)
5	Mildly frail (limited dependence in IADL)
6	Moderately frail (help needed with ADL and IADL)
7	Severely frail (completely dependent in ADL, or terminally ill)

Reprinted from Rockwood K, Song X, MacKnight C, et al. A global clinical measure of fitness and frailty in elderly people. *Can Med Assoc J.* 2005;173(5):489-495, with permission.

What role can the assessment of frailty play into preoperative decision-making?

Given its association with postsurgical morbidity and mortality, frailty can be incorporated into preoperative assessment to help guide decision-making.

A 2018 retrospective analysis of the ACS-NSQIP database evaluated frailty in a cohort of 984,550 patients from 2005 to 2012 who had undergone inpatient general, vascular, orthopedic, thoracic, or cardiac surgery.[4] Patients were excluded if they were under the age of 18 years or did not have enough data obtained to measure frailty. Frailty was measured by the RAI-A, and patients were stratified by quintiles (lowest quintile defined as RAI-A ≤10; highest quintile defined as RAI-A >40). Surgical procedures were categorized as low-risk (≤1% mortality risk) versus high-risk (>1% mortality risk).

Outcomes included major complications (including postoperative infections, pulmonary embolism, bleeding requiring transfusion, stroke) and the occurrence of failure to rescue (death after potentially avoidable surgical complication).

---

[4]Shah R, et al. Association of frailty with failure to rescue after low-risk and high-risk inpatient surgery. *JAMA Surg.* 2018;153(5):e180214.

The average age of patients in the study was 58 years. RAI-A score was associated in a dose-dependent manner with major complications and failure to rescue in both low-risk and high-risk surgical procedures. Major complication rates after low-risk surgery were 3.2% in the lowest RAI-A quintile and 36.4% in the highest RAI-A quintile ($P < .001$ across all quintiles). After high-risk surgery, major complication rates were 13.5% and 54.4% for the lowest and highest RAI-A quintiles, respectively ($P < .001$ across all quintiles).

Similarly, failure to rescue increased with increasing RAI-A and number of complications. Among patients undergoing high-risk procedures and experiencing one major complication, patients in the four highest RAI-A quintiles were more likely to experience failure to rescue compared to patients in the lowest RAI-A quintile. For example, patients with RAI-A >40 were more likely to experience failure to rescue (OR 18.4, 95% CI 15.7-21.4; P-value not reported). Similar findings were observed for low-risk procedures. Notably, the association between RAI-A and failure to rescue decreased with increasing number of complications, suggesting that complications may attenuate the effect of frailty. Study caveats include retrospective design and lack of use of RAI-A threshold to dichotomize between frail versus nonfrail patients.

Together with your surgical colleague, you express your concerns about the patient's frailty to her and her family. After careful discussion of risks and benefits, they elect to undergo surgical intervention. She tolerates the procedure and does well postoperatively prior to discharge to a skilled nursing facility.

You are paged by the nurse to talk with the family of another patient on your service, a 90-year-old man admitted from home several days ago with pneumonia. The patient's family has arrived at the hospital and would like to discuss and receive an update on the patient's discharge plan.

As you walk to the patient's room, you review his case with the medical student on your service. You review that the patient's medical history is notable for mild dementia and chronic obstructive pulmonary disease (COPD), and that despite being independent in transfers, he is mostly wheelchair bound at baseline and receives caregiver services daily for assistance with cooking, housework, transportation, and bathing. In teaching the medical student on your service about frailty, you determine that the patient is moderately frail based on a CSHA-CFS score of 6.

What is the impact of frailty on hospitalized patients' hospital and postdischarge course?

Frail patients can be at increased risk for in-hospital mortality and new nursing home placement. Because frail patients can have slower recovery trajectories and greater discharge needs, they may benefit from early physical therapy evaluation during hospitalization.

An analysis conducted in 2015 addressed this question by evaluating the effect of frailty among 2125 adults admitted to geriatricians at a single tertiary referral hospital in Australia.[5] Frailty was defined using the CSHA-CFS (Table 28.1). Outcomes included in-hospital mortality, new nursing home placement, and hospital length of stay (LOS).

Compared to nonfrail patients, severely frail patients were more likely to experience in-hospital mortality (OR 2.97, 95% CI 2.11-4.17; *P* < .001) and new nursing home placement (OR 1.60, 95% 1.14-2.24; *P* = .006), and had a lower probability of discharge, i.e., longer LOS (HR 0.87, 95% 0.81-0.93; *P* < .001). Caveats include single-site design and limitations on generalizability to patients cared for by nongeriatrician generalists.

A 2017 retrospective analysis evaluated the association between frailty and outcomes among 493 patients ≥75 years of age admitted to the geriatric service in a tertiary teaching hospital in the United Kingdom.[6] Frailty was defined using an expanded version of the Clinical Frailty Scale (CFS), with a spectrum of functional decline ranging from a score of 1 (physically fit) to 9 (terminally ill). Patients were categorized as nonfrail (CFS score <5), moderately frail (CFS score 5-6), or severely frail (CFS score 7-8). Patients with CFS scores of 9 were excluded to avoid bias from terminal illness. The primary outcome was recovery trajectory, which was evaluated by trended function scores at baseline, admission, and discharge, with function evaluated via the modified Rankin Scale (mRS). The mRS ranges from 1 (no significant disability despite symptoms) to 6 (dead), with a score of 5 reflecting severe disability or a bedridden, incontinent state requiring constant nursing attention/care. LOS was also evaluated.

Recovery trajectory varied by the extent of patient frailty (Figure). Mean mRS for nonfrail patients trended from 1.8 (95% CI 1.7-2.0) at

[5]Basic D, Shanley C. Frailty in an older inpatient population: using the clinical frailty scale to predict patient outcomes. *J Aging Health*. 2015;27(4):670-685.

[6]Hartley P, et al. Clinical frailty and functional trajectories in hospitalized older adults: a retrospective observational study. *Geriatr Gerontol Int*. 2017;17:1063-1068.

baseline to 3.3 (95% CI 3.1-3.5) at hospital admission and 2.2 (95% CI 2.0-2.3) at discharge. In comparison, mRS for moderately frail patients trended from 2.9 (95% CI 2.8-3.0) at baseline to 4.0 (95% CI 3.8-4.1) at admission and 3.2 (95% CI 3.1-3.3) at discharge, while the mean mRS for severely frail patients trend from 3.5 (95% CI 3.3-3.6) at baseline to 4.3 (95% CI 4.1-4.4) at admission and 3.7 (95% CI 3.6-3.9) at discharge. The mean LOS for severely frail patients was 17.5 days compared to 9.1 days for nonfrail patients ($P < .001$). Study caveats include retrospective observational study design and 20% mortality during hospitalization among severely frail patients.

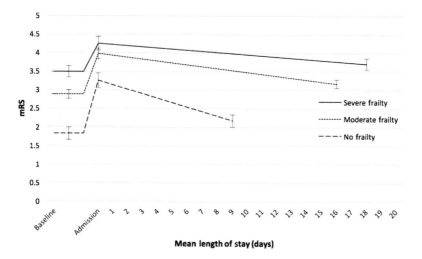

Mean length of stay (days)

Another 2017 observational analysis[7] conducted at the same tertiary teaching hospital evaluated the association between early physical therapy and outcomes among 1003 hospital admissions of patients ≥75 years of age. Frailty was assessed using the 9-point CFS, with a median score of 6 across the study cohort. After excluding patients not assessed by physical therapy during their hospitalization, eligible patients were dichotomized into those receiving early (within 24 hours of hospital admission) versus late (after the first 24 hours hospitalized) evaluation by physical therapy. Outcomes included hospital LOS, change in mobility between admission and discharge (assessed by the Elder Mobility Score, EMS, a 20-point scale used to evaluate function in frail older patients), and need

[7]Hartley PJ, et al. Earlier physical therapy input is associated with a reduced length of hospital stay and reduced care needs on discharge in frail older inpatients: an observational study. *J Geriatr Phys Ther.* 2019;42(2):E7-E14.

for new formal care package (i.e., care provided by an external agency) or postdischarge institutionalization (i.e., discharge to care institution among patients admitted from home). Discharge to usual residence was also evaluated.

Pairwise comparisons were conducted for outcomes between the early and late evaluation groups. Additionally, among patients admitted from home (rather than nursing home or institutional facility), Cox proportional hazards regression was used to evaluate the association between early physical therapy evaluation and discharge home. Covariates included in regression analysis included patient demographics, mobility at admission, and Charlson Comorbidity Index.

Patients receiving early evaluation had shorter median hospital LOS (6.7 vs. 10.0 days; $P < .001$) and less need for new formal care package (20.3% vs. 27.0%; $P = .02$) but did not exhibit differential changes in mobility (median change of 0 for both early and late evaluation groups; $P = .83$) or in need for institutionalization (4.1% vs. 6.7%; $P = .073$). Discharge to usual residence was more common among early evaluation patients (HR 1.34, 95% CI, 1.16-1.55; $P < .001$). Study limitations include single-center observational design, and the fact that assessment by physical therapy did not involve evaluation of whether suggested interventions were ultimately implemented.

You recommend early physical therapy consult and talk with the patient and his family about the possibility that he may need a higher level of care at discharge. He improves clinically with antibiotics and is able to discharge home with 24-hour supervision 2 days following admission.

KEY LEARNING POINTS

1. Numerous instruments have been developed to evaluate frailty in hospitalized surgical and medical patients.
2. Frailty can be incorporated into preoperative assessment to help guide surgical decision-making.
3. Frail patients can have higher risk for several adverse outcomes and may benefit from early physical therapy evaluation during hospitalization.

COMMUNICATION IN ACADEMIC HOSPITAL MEDICINE

Leah Marcotte, MD,
Joshua M. Liao, MD, MSc

It is your first day on an inpatient teaching service with a third-year internal medicine resident, two interns, and two third-year medical students. You meet your team to begin clinical patient rounds, and the resident asks how you would like to round on patients—inside or outside the room and with or without the patient's nurse.

What are the potential benefits of interprofessional bedside rounding for clinical team members?

Interprofessional bedside rounds can improve perceptions of communication, coordination, and teamwork among physician and nurse team members.

A 2014 single-site study[1] evaluated this question by conducting a cross-sectional survey of three groups of clinicians (hospital-based attending physicians, housestaff physicians, and nurses) at an academic teaching hospital with existing experience in interdisciplinary bedside rounds. These rounds were defined as encounters involving at least two physicians and either a nurse or other team member in which a patient's case presentation was discussed either in or outside the room followed by a bedside discussion in which the patient was encouraged to participate and ask questions. The survey was conducted using an instrument designed for the study based on prior literature and centered on

---

[1]Gonzalo JD, et al. Bedside interprofessional rounds: perceptions of benefits and barriers by internal medicine nursing staff, attending physicians, and housestaff physicians. *J Hosp Med*. 2014;9(10):646-651.

five domains related to the putative benefits of interprofessional bedside rounds (patient factors; a composite of communication, coordination, and teamwork; education; efficiency/process; and patient outcomes) and four domains related to barriers to such rounds (patient factors; clinician factors; systems-related issues; time-related issues). Pairwise statistical tests were used to compare survey responses between clinician groups, and a Spearman rank test (r) was used to evaluate the correlation in rank ordering of stated benefits and barriers by the clinician group.

Survey response rate was 87% (149/171). There was high correlation between domain rankings for hospital-based physicians, housestaff physicians, and nurses (r = 0.92, $P < .001$). Benefits of interprofessional bedside rounds that were ranked most highly related to communication, coordination, and teamwork, while the lowest ranked benefits related to efficiency/process and rounding outcomes (e.g., "timeliness of consultations"). For each survey item related to benefits, nurses reported more favorable ratings than hospital-based and housestaff physicians. The greatest perceived barriers to interprofessional bedside rounds related to issues of time (e.g., "nursing staff have limited time"), compared to the least perceived barriers which pertained to patient factors (e.g., "patient lack of comfort") and clinician factors (e.g., physicians lacking "bedside skills"). The three clinician groups possessed moderate correlation in rank ordering of interprofessional bedside rounds barriers (r = 0.62-0.82 across the three groups). Study caveats include single-site design and lack of psychometric instrument testing.

While more work is needed to understand the full effects of bedside rounding,[2] ACGME regulations[3] include the expectation that residents work in interprofessional teams to improve safety and quality of care in an environment that optimizes effective communication with all team members.

You finish patient rounds and remind the resident that it is time for you both to attend daily interdisciplinary rounds. Having never heard of these rounds before, the medical students inquire about their role in patient care.

[2]Gamp M, et al. Effect of bedside vs. non-bedside patient case presentation during ward rounds: a systematic review and meta-analysis. *J Gen Intern Med*. 2019;34(3):447-457.
[3]Accreditation Council for Graduate Medical Education. *Common Program Requirements*. Available at: https://www.acgme.org/Portals/0/PFAssets/ProgramRequirements/CPRResidency2019.pdf. Accessed September 14, 2019.

What are the potential benefits of structured interdisciplinary rounds (SIDRs) to patient care?

SIDR can be associated with perceptions of stronger collaboration, communication, and safety climate, as well as fewer adverse events.

A study conducted in 2011[4] at a single academic medical center evaluated this question by implementing SIDR via a structured daily meeting between resident physicians, pharmacists, social workers, and case managers assigned to the care of patients on a medical unit. Another unit in the hospital where SIDR was not implemented served as a control. Newly admitted patients on the intervention unit were discussed via a structured communication tool designed by the interdisciplinary care team (Table 29.1). Patients on the control unit were discussed without the communication tool. Clinicians and team members on both the intervention and control units were surveyed using questions adapted from prior studies about the quality of communication and collaboration as well as about the patient safety climate. Multivariable regression, adjusted for factors such as patient demographics, medical complexity, case-mix, admission source, hospitalist as attending physician, and payer, was used to evaluate length of stay (LOS) and hospital costs as other study outcomes.

Survey response rate was 92% (147/159 eligible respondents). Because of small numbers, data from social workers, case managers, and pharmacists were excluded from analysis. Nurses on the intervention unit rated the quality of collaboration and communication (74% rating it as high vs. 44% of nurses on the control unit; $P = .02$) and teamwork (mean score 84 vs. 74 on the control unit; $P = .005$) more highly than nurses on the control unit. In contrast, there were no differences observed in resident ratings about the quality of collaboration and communication (91% rating it as high vs. 88% of residents on the control unit; $P = .57$) or safety climate ratings across all providers (mean score 77 vs. 75 on the control unit: $P = .90$), along with adjusted LOS and cost of hospitalization. Caveats included single-site design, imbalance in the proportion of patients with hospitalist attendings between intervention and control units, and lack of clinical outcomes.

---

[4]O'Leary KJ, et al. Improving teamwork: Impact of structured interdisciplinary rounds on a medical teaching unit. *J Gen Intern Med*. 2010; 25(8):826-832.

TABLE 29.1

SIDR Communication Tool

Overall plan of care
- Diagnosis?
- Patient's chief concern?
- Tests today?
- Procedures today?
- Medication changes today?
- Medication issues?
- Consulting services?
- Expected discharge date?

Discharge plans
- Telemetry needed?
- Discharge needs?
  - ▪ Placement?
  - ▪ Home health needs?
  - ▪ Transportation?

Patient safety
- On VTE prophylaxis?
- Can central lines be discontinued (including PICCs)?
- Can Foley catheter bed be continued
- Can we reduce fall risk?
- Can we reduce pressure ulcer risk?

PICC, peripherally inserted central catheter; SIDR, structured interdisciplinary rounds; VTE, venous thromboembolism.

Reprinted by permission from Springer Nature: *Gen Intern Med.* Improving teamwork: Impact of structured interdisciplinary rounds on a medical teaching unit. O'Leary KJ, et al., 2010.

A subsequent study conducted at the same academic medical center in 2011[5] used a similar design of intervention versus control unit to evaluate the relationship between the same SIDR intervention on adverse events as study outcomes. Adverse events were defined as injuries due to medical care rather than illness and were identified via medical record abstraction and application of screening criteria used in prior research on a randomly selected subset of 555 patients. Physician reviewers independently rated the presence and preventability of identified adverse events before coming to consensus (κ 0.78 and 1 for presence and preventability of adverse events, respectively).

---

[5]O'Leary KJ, et al. Structured interdisciplinary rounds in a medical teaching unit: improving patient safety. *Arch Intern Med.* 2011;171(7):678-684.

The adverse event rate was lower after implementation of SIDR (3.9 per 100 patient-days) in concurrent (7.2 per 100 patient-days, RR 0.54; $P = .005$) and historical (7.7 per 100 patient-days, RR 0.51; $P = .001$) comparisons to control units. The rate of preventable adverse events was also lower in the intervention unit after implementation of SIDR in concurrent (RR 0.27; $P = .002$) and historical (RR 0.37; $P = .02$) comparisons to the control unit. Study caveats include retrospective design and use of chart review to identify adverse events.

Despite the limitations of these studies, interdisciplinary rounds are implemented widely in hospitals. Though format and structure vary across institutions, such rounds are promoted as a means for potentially improving quality, safety, and other outcomes by groups such as the Institute for Healthcare Improvement.[6]

> You touch base and run the list with the resident in the early evening, and you determine together that the team has completed all of its tasks for the day. The resident asks if you have any specific input for her pass off to the nighttime resident.

What measures can be used to help reduce medical errors related to change of shift pass off?

Structured approaches to communicating information during pass off, including those that incorporate the SIGNOUT mnemonic or I-PASS bundle, can reduce medical errors and preventable adverse events.

This question was addressed in a 2013 prospective pre–post study [7] conducted on two units at a single US pediatric academic medical center. Resident physicians were trained in a multifaceted pass-off intervention that consisted of (1) formal communication training, (2) introduction of the SIGNOUT mnemonic for verbal pass off (Table 29.2), and (3) implementation of a new pass-off structure including periodic oversight by chief residents or attending physicians and

---

[6]Institute for Healthcare Improvement. *How-to Guide: Multidisciplinary Rounds.* Available at: http://www.ihi.org/resources/Pages/Tools/HowtoGuideMultidisciplinaryRounds.aspx. Accessed September 14, 2019.

[7]Starmer AJ, et al. Rates of medical errors and preventable adverse events among hospitalized children following implementation of a resident handoff bundle. *J Am Med Assoc.* 2013;310(21):2262-2270.

TABLE 29.2

SIGNOUT Format for Oral Communication

	Mnemonic	Sample sign-out
S	Sick or DNR? (highlight sick or unstable patients, identify DNR/DNI patients)	OK, this is our sickest patient, and he is full code.
I	Identifying data (name, age, gender, diagnosis)	Mr. Jones is a 77-year-old gentleman with a right middle lobe pneumonia.
G	General hospital course	He came in a week ago hypoxic and hypotensive but improved rapidly with IV levofloxacin.
N	New events of day	Today he developed a temp of 39.5°C and his white count went from 8 to 14. We got a portable chest x-ray, which was improved from admission, took out his Foley and sent blood and urine cultures. U/A was negative but his IV site looked a little red so we started vancomycin.
O	Overall health status/clinical condition	Right now he is satting 98% on 2 L nasal cannula and is afebrile.
U	Upcoming possibilities with plan, rationale	If he becomes persistently febrile or starts to drop his pressures, start normal saline at 125 cc/h and have a low threshold for calling the ICU to take a look at him because of concern for sepsis.
T	Tasks to complete overnight with plan, rationale	I would like you to look in on him around midnight and make sure his vitals and examination are unchanged. I do not expect any blood culture results back tonight, so there is no need to follow those up.
?	Any questions?	Any questions?

DNI, Do Not Intubate; DNR, Do Not Resuscitate.

Reprinted by permission from Springer Nature. *J Gen Intern Med.* Development and implementation of an oral sign-out skills curriculum. Horwitz LI, Moin T, Green ML, 2007.

incorporating integrated intern and senior resident pass offs. On one patient care unit, an electronic medical record-integrated pass-off tool that incorporated structured data fields (e.g., "Patient Summary", "Contingency Planning") was also used. Primary outcomes included medical error and preventable adverse event rates (based on systematic surveillance, which included review of medical charts and reports from clinicians). Secondary outcomes included omissions in written pass offs (based on investigator review of pass-off documents and determination of major changes in 14 predefined data elements such as patient identifiers, code status, reason for admission, patient summary, contingency plans, etc.).

Compared to the preintervention period, medical error rates decreased in the postintervention period (from 34/100 admissions, 95% CI 27-40, to 18/100 admissions, 95% CI 15-22; $P < .001$). Similarly, the rate of preventable adverse events decreased postintervention (from 3/100 admissions, 95% CI 2-5, to 2/100 admissions, 95% CI 0.5-2; $P = .04$). The intervention was associated with fewer written pass-off omissions, particularly among participants from the clinical unit utilizing the electronic medical record–integrated tool (reductions in omissions for 11 of 14 predefined data elements compared to the preintervention period, $P < .05$). Study caveats include single-site scope and focus on pediatric patients.

This study led directly to the development of the I-PASS pass-off bundle, which was subsequently tested in a 2014 multicenter study[8] conducted among pediatric resident physicians across 10,740 admissions at nine North American hospitals. The I-PASS bundle consisted of multiple components, including formal communication training, a mnemonic for verbal pass off (Table 29.3), 1-hour role-playing and simulation session, a computer module, and direct-observation and feedback tools for attending physicians. Coprimary outcomes were medical errors and preventable adverse events, which were evaluated via active surveillance by a research nurse and subsequently reviewed and categorized by blinded physicians either as an adverse event, near miss or error with little potential for harm, or incident not reflecting medical error or an adverse event. Secondary outcomes included nonpreventable adverse events.

The bundle led to reductions in both medical errors (25/100 admissions pre intervention vs. 19/100 admissions postintervention) and preventable adverse events (5/100 admissions vs. 3/100 admissions) ($P < .001$ for both). The nonpreventable adverse event rate did not change between the pre- and postintervention periods (3 vs. 3/100 admissions; $P = .79$). Caveats include pre–post design, variation in

---

[8]Starmer AJ, et al. Changes in medical errors after implementation of a handoff program. *N Engl J Med*. 2014;371:1803-1812.

TABLE 29.3

I-PASS Mnemonic

I	Illness Severity	• Stable, "watcher," unstable
P	Patient summary	• Summary events • Events leading up to admission • Hospital course • Ongoing assessment • Plan
A	Action list	• To-do list • Time line and ownership
S	Situation awareness and contingency planning	• Know what is going on • Plan for what might happen
S	Synthesis by the receiver	• Receiver summarizes what was heard • Asks questions • Restates key action/to-do items

Reprinted from Starmer AJ, et al. I-pass, a mnemonic to standardize verbal handoffs. *Pediatrics.* 2012;129(2):201-204, with permission from American Academy of Pediatrics.

baseline error rates, and heterogeneity in which study sites exhibited reductions in study outcomes (no significant changes in error rates at three of nine sites for unclear reasons).

ACGME Common Program Requirements[9] stipulate that training programs and institutions must ensure and monitor structured pass-off processes for patient safety and care continuity.

You review the I-PASS mnemonic and other aspects of the bundle with the resident and observe her pass off the care of your team's patients to the night resident.

On rounds the next morning, you and your team plan to discharge an elderly patient who has had a complicated course to a skilled nursing facility (SNF). The intern taking care of the patient asks if there is anything he can do to optimize the patient's transition.

---

[9]Accreditation Council for Graduate Medical Education. *Common Program Requirements.* Available at: https://www.acgme.org/Portals/0/PFAssets/ProgramRequirements/CPRResidency2019.pdf. Accessed September 14, 2019.

How can planned interdisciplinary communication between the inpatient and SNF teams improve outcomes in older adults?

Direct communication between the interdisciplinary inpatient and SNF teams may be beneficial in reducing 30-day readmissions, SNF LOS, and total costs of care for older adults discharged to SNFs.

A prospective cohort study at a single academic medical center examined this question by evaluating how outcomes for 1059 patients discharged from hospital to SNF were affected by Extension for Community Health Outcomes-Care Transitions (ECHO-CT), a videoconference intervention between the inpatient and SNF teams.[10] The ECHO-CT intervention consisted of a 90-minute weekly videoconference, during which each patient was discussed for up to 10 minutes by inpatient (discharging inpatient physicians, pharmacist, social worker, hospitalist facilitator, project manager, as well as often patients' primary care physicians) and SNF (physicians, nurses, physical therapists) teams. Each discussion was documented in the patient's medical record. Patients receiving ECHO-CT were compared to control patients based on SNF-level matching (i.e., SNFs participating in ECHO-CT matched based on quality and size to nonparticipating SNFs). Study outcomes included 30-day readmission rate, 30-day mortality, SNF LOS, and total costs of care. Multivariate regression, adjusted for factors such as demographics and case mix, was used to analyze the relationship between the ECHO-CT intervention and outcomes.

In multivariate analysis, patients in the intervention group had lower 30-day readmission rates (OR 0.57, 95% CI 0.34-0.96; $P = .034$), SNF LOS (mean estimate difference between groups of 5.52 days, 95% CI 9.61-1.43; $P = .01$), and total healthcare cost (mean between group difference of $2602.19 per patient, 95% CI $1070.48-$4133.90; $P < .001$) than patients in the control group. The adjusted 30-day mortality rate did not differ between groups (OR 0.38 95% CI 0.11-1.24; $P = .11$). Caveats include prospective cohort and single-centered design, nonrandomization of participating SNFs, and limited generalizability due to implementation of ECHO-CT within an accountable care organization.

---

[10]Moore AB, et al. Improving transitions to postacute care for elderly patients using a novel video-conferencing program: ECHO-care transitions. *Am J Med*. 2017;130(10):1199-1204.

Upon discharging the patient, you and the senior resident contact the attending physician at the SNF to review the patient's hospital course and discuss potential issues to address during the care transition.

KEY LEARNING POINTS

1. Interprofessional bedside rounds can improve perceptions about communication, coordination, and teamwork among clinical team members.
2. Structured interdisciplinary rounds can be associated with perceptions of stronger collaboration, communication, and safer care.
3. Structured approaches to communicating information during pass off can reduce medical errors and preventable adverse events.
4. Direct communication between the inpatient and SNF teams may be beneficial in improving outcomes among patients discharged from hospitals to SNFs.

END-OF-LIFE CARE

Zahir Kanjee, MD, MPH,
Cindy Lien, MD

You admit an 88-year-old man with advanced dementia after his fourth bout of aspiration pneumonia this year. He is stabilized and improves with antibiotics. Swallowing evaluation confirms progressive dysphagia. His daughter is his health care proxy and asks about placing a percutaneous endoscopic gastrostomy (PEG) tube for artificial feeding to prevent aspiration and improve his mortality risk.

Does PEG placement improve survival in patients with advanced dementia?

PEG placement does not prolong life in this setting.

A large retrospective study assessed the association between PEG placement and survival in 36,492 patients with advanced dementia.[1] Patients with a diagnosis of dementia based on the Minimum Data Set (a national nursing home database) were eligible for inclusion at the point of severe deficits in decision-making capacity with total dependence for eating, determined from their Cognitive Performance Scale, a validated dementia functional score. Patients were excluded if they were comatose or had received PEG feeding in the previous 6 months. Multivariable survival analysis utilized inverse probability weighting (to address selection bias) and controlled for demographic variables,

---

[1]Teno JM, et al. Does feeding tube insertion and its timing improve survival? *J Am Geriatr Soc.* 2012;60(10):1918-1921.

advanced care plans, comorbidities, dietary and nutritional variables, functional status, and models of mortality. PEG placement was not associated with an increase in survival (HR 1.03, 95% CI 0.94-1.13; P-value not reported). Study caveats include the observational and retrospective nature and use of administrative data.

These findings are in line with a 2009 Cochrane review of enteral tube feeding among elderly adults with advanced dementia.[2] The review included experimental and observational studies comparing tube feeding (either PEG or nasogastric) to usual care/no intervention. Studies were included if >50% of patients were suffering from dementia. Patients were also required to be ≥50 years old with nutritional problems or difficulty eating or swallowing, with cognitive impairment assessed by any validated tool. There were two primary outcomes: mortality and quality of life. Secondary outcomes included nutritional endpoints (including body mass index [BMI], weight, and albumin), healing of pressure sores, and adverse outcomes like aspiration pneumonia and local or systemic complications.

The review included seven observational studies, each of which was deemed at high risk of bias. No studies found an improvement in survival associated with tube feeding after adjustment for comorbidity, while two studies showed an increase in mortality with tube feeding. There were no studies addressing quality of life, and several did not report on key adverse outcomes. Evidence for effects on pressure ulcers was mixed. One study found a higher rate of aspiration pneumonia in tube-fed patients. Limitations of this review include the use of observational studies, individual study bias, and inclusion of studies with small sample sizes and/or nondementia-related cognitive impairment.

Consistent with these findings, the AGS[3] and the AAHPM[4] do not recommend percutaneous tube feeding in advanced dementia.

---

[2]Sampson EL, et al. Enteral tube feeding for older people with advanced dementia. *Cochrane Database Syst Rev.* 2009;(2):CD007209.

[3]American Geriatrics Society Ethics Committee and Clinical Practice and Models of Care Committee. American Geriatrics Society feeding tubes in advanced dementia position statement. *J Am Geriatr Soc.* 2014;62(8):1590-1593.

[4]American Academy of Hospice and Palliative Medicine. *Five Things Physicians and Patients Should Question.* American Board of Internal Medicine Foundation. Available at: http://www.choosingwisely.org/societies/american-academy-of-hospice-and-palliative-medicine/. Accessed December 13, 2018.

You meet with the patient's daughter to discuss her question about PEG placement. Using a shared-decision-making approach, you explore the patient's goals and values before discussing the clinical implications of PEG placement in advanced dementia. You ultimately advise against PEG placement and the daughter agrees with your recommendation.

Several weeks later, the patient is readmitted with a submassive pulmonary embolism. Soon after, he clinically decompensates and suffers a cardiac arrest. Cardiopulmonary resuscitation (CPR) is immediately begun in accordance with his advance directives. A colleague takes over the acute management as you step out to inform the patient's daughter, who is just arriving on the floor. You inform her of these events and wonder whether you should invite her to observe resuscitation efforts.

What are the potential effects of permitting a patient's family member to observe CPR?

Family members who are invited to be present during a patient's CPR have lower subsequent rates of posttraumatic stress disorder (PTSD), depression, and complicated grief. Hospital family presence policies are not associated with harmful effects on CPR efforts or patient outcomes.

Investigators in France randomized 15 prehospital emergency medical service teams (including an emergency medicine physician) to either an intervention or usual-care strategy for all adults with cardiac arrest undergoing resuscitation at home from October 2009 to November 2011.[5] Teams in the intervention group used a communication guide to routinely and explicitly invite a single adult first-degree relative to witness CPR. The usual-care teams did not specifically invite relatives to witness CPR but permitted it if requested. The primary outcome was the prevalence of PTSD symptoms (using the Impact of Event Scale as assessed by a blinded psychologist) among the 570 selected family members at 90 days after resuscitation. Those who could not complete the assessment due to emotional distress were deemed also to have PTSD symptoms. Secondary outcomes included rates of anxiety and depression (based on the Hospital Anxiety and Depression Scale, HADS),

---

[5]Jabre P, et al. Family presence during cardiopulmonary resuscitation. *N Engl J Med.* 2013;368(11):1008-1018.

resuscitation efforts (such as duration of CPR or number of shocks), medical team emotional stress (on a visual analogue scale), and medico-legal claims. To assess the impact of family members actually observing CPR, several outcomes were also analyzed based on whether the CPR was witnessed or unwitnessed regardless of patient group assignment.

The rate of PTSD symptoms was higher among family members of patients resuscitated by the usual-care group (OR 1.7, 95% CI 1.2-2.5; P = .004). Symptoms of anxiety (P < .001) but not depression (P = .13) were also higher among family members of patients resuscitated by the usual-care group. Family members witnessing CPR was associated with lower rates of symptoms of PTSD (P = .01), anxiety (P < .001), and depression (P = .009). There were no differences between witnessed and unwitnessed episodes in terms of duration of CPR, number of shocks, survival to hospital admission, or medical team stress. There were no medicolegal claims in any of the cases at median 20 months follow-up.

In a longer-term 1-year follow-up study of the same population,[6] family members of patients treated by the intervention group teams had a lower prevalence of PTSD (P = .02) and depression (P = .003) symptoms as well as complicated grief (P = .005).

Caveats of these studies include limited generalizability to in-hospital arrests and non-French settings.

A 2015 observational study assessed the effects of a hospital policy permitting family presence during resuscitation on patient-level outcomes among 41,568 patients with cardiac arrest at 252 hospitals participating in a nationwide registry. Patients were included if they were ≥18 years of age and had cardiac arrest. Patients were excluded if they had an implantable defibrillator or if their arrest occurred in an undocumented or procedural (such as a delivery room, cardiac catheterization lab, or electrophysiology suite) area of the hospital. The primary outcomes were return of spontaneous circulation (ROSC) and survival to discharge. Secondary outcomes included favorable neurologic status at discharge (no or only moderate disability, as opposed to severe disability, coma or vegetative state, and brain death), time to defibrillation, and duration of resuscitation. Given expected skew of findings between those who survived and those who did not, a number of these outcomes were examined separately in survivors and nonsurvivors. Linear and logistic regression models were adjusted for variables such as initial arrest rhythm, patient demographics, comorbidities, presenting illness

---

[6]Jabre P, et al. Offering the opportunity for family to be present during cardiopulmonary resuscitation: 1-year assessment. *Intensive Care Med.* 2014;40(7):981-987.

category, whether arrest was witnessed or unwitnessed, time from identification of pulselessness to compressions, and hospital characteristics
(such as location, size, and teaching status).

Rates of ROSC (RR 1.02, 95% CI 0.98-1.06; no *P*-value reported),
survival to discharge (RR 1.05, 95% CI 0.95-1.15; no *P*-value reported),
and discharge with favorable neurologic status (RR = 0.97, 95% CI
0.92-1.02; no *P*-value reported) were not associated with the existence
of a policy on family presence during resuscitation. There were no differences in time to mean defibrillation (mean difference 0.32 minutes;
P = .05) or median number of shocks delivered (*P* = .45). Among nonsurvivors, patients in hospitals with family presence policies received a
longer median duration of resuscitation (mean difference 1.4 minutes,
95% CI 0.08-2.7; *P* = .04). Caveats include that this study tested the
effect of the presence of a policy rather than routine implementation
of that policy, that the exposure of interest was at the hospital and not
patient level, the lack of information about the presence of family members at resuscitation, as well as a large number of secondary outcomes
(which increases the risk of a chance finding).

> You invite the patient's daughter to witness resuscitation efforts and
> she accepts. The patient unfortunately never regains spontaneous
> circulation and dies. His daughter is devastated but expresses grati-
> tude for your care. She accepts a visit from the hospital chaplain. The
> social worker also meets with her and provides information on local
> bereavement support services.
>
> Also on your service is a previously healthy 67-year-old woman
> who presented with cough and weight loss and subsequently under-
> went biopsy after pulmonary and liver masses were found on imaging
> studies. Her biopsy results confirm a diagnosis of metastatic non–
> small-cell lung cancer (NSCLC). She and the consulting oncologist
> are considering options for a treatment regimen as an outpatient.
> You wonder if concurrent palliative care referral would be helpful.

What are the possible effects of early palliative care referral for patients with newly diagnosed advanced cancer?

Early palliative care referral for advanced cancer can lead to improvements in quality of life for patients and short-term reductions in distress
for their caregivers. In some cases, early palliative care is associated with
longer survival.

In a 2010 nonblinded trial[7] conducted at a large US academic medical center, 151 patients with metastatic NSCLC diagnosed within the last 8 weeks were randomized to usual oncologic care with or without early palliative care. Patients were included if they had adequate functional status (Eastern Cooperative Oncology Group, ECOG, score ≤2, indicating <50% of the day spent in bed) and were excluded if they were already receiving palliative care. The early palliative care group met with palliative specialists within 3 weeks of randomization and then at least once per month afterward until the time of death. Usual-care patients were referred to palliative care only when requested by the patient, family, or treatment team. The primary outcome was the change in quality of life from baseline to 12 weeks (defined by Trial Outcome Index, TOI, a summation of physical and functional scales). Secondary outcomes included depression (assessed by the HADS and the Patient Health Questionnaire 9, PHQ-9) and mortality at study completion. Compared to the usual-care group, which experienced decreases in quality of life, the early palliative care group demonstrated moderate improvements (between-group difference in TOI 6.0, 95% CI 1.5-10.4; $P = .009$). The early palliative care group was less likely to be depressed by PHQ-9 criteria (4% vs. 17%; $P = .04$) despite equal rates of new antidepressant prescription. The early palliative care group had longer median survival (11.6 vs. 8.9 months; $P = .02$).

A subsequent randomized controlled trial at the same academic medical center evaluated the effects of early palliative care among family members of patients with newly diagnosed advanced lung and gastrointestinal cancers.[8] Patients ≥18 years of age were included if they were within 8 weeks of a new diagnosis of an incurable lung or noncolorectal gastrointestinal cancer, had never received treatment for metastatic disease, and had adequate performance status (ECOG ≤2). Patients were excluded if they were already receiving palliative care or had significant psychiatric comorbidity. Eligible patients were asked to name an adult (≥18 years of age) caregiver they anticipated would be present with them at clinic visits. A total of 275 caregivers were enrolled in this trial.

Patients in the early palliative care group received an outpatient palliative care visit within 4 weeks and then monthly afterward until

[7]Temel JS, et al. Early palliative care for patients with metastatic non-small-cell lung cancer. *N Engl J Med.* 2010;363(8):733-742.
[8]El-Jawahri A, et al. Effects of early integrated palliative care on caregivers of patients with lung and gastrointestinal cancer: a randomized clinical trial. *Oncologist.* 2017;22(12):1528-1534.

death, as well as routine inpatient palliative care consultation when admitted to the academic medical center. Patients in the usual-care group were referred to palliative care only if specifically requested by the patient, caregiver, or oncology team. Key outcomes included caregiver distress (using the HADS) and quality of life (using the Medical Health Outcomes Survey-Short Form, SF-36). Assessments were performed at 12 and 24 weeks, and all values were adjusted for baseline scores.

Caregivers of patients in the early palliative care group demonstrated lower distress (adjusted mean difference between the early palliative care and control groups −1.45, 95% CI −2.76 to −0.15; P = .029) at week 12 but there were no differences at 24 weeks (P = .279). There were no differences in quality of life at 12 (P = .183) or 24 weeks (P = .669).

Caveats for each of these two studies include generalizability concerns due to their single-centered nature and racially homogeneous (primarily Caucasian) patients. The latter study is also limited by measurement of multiple outcomes at multiple timepoints without a clearly specified primary outcome.

Finally, a 2014 cluster-randomized study conducted at 24 cancer clinics affiliated with a single Canadian tertiary academic oncology center assessed the effects of early palliative care in a broader range of advanced cancers.[9] Adult (≥18 years of age) patients were included if they had stage III or IV solid tumor cancer, life expectancy of 6 to 24 months (per their oncologist's assessment), and adequate performance status (ECOG≤2). Patients in the early palliative care group received a clinic visit within 1 month and monthly thereafter. The usual-care group received palliative care only as requested.

The primary outcome was quality of life (based on the Functional Assessment of Chronic Illness Therapy—Spiritual Well-Being scale, FACIT-Sp) at 3 months. Secondary outcomes included FACIT-Sp scores at 4 months as well as quality of life at the end of life (based on the Quality of Life at the End of Life scale, QUAL-E), symptoms (based on the Edmonton Symptom Assessment System, ESAS), and patient satisfaction with care (based on the family satisfaction with advanced cancer scale, FAMCARE-P16) at 3 and 4 months.

There was no difference in the quality of life between groups at 3 months (adjusted difference of 3.56, 95% CI −0.27 to 7.40; P = .07), but there was at 4 months (adjusted difference of 6.44, 95% CI

[9]Zimmerman C, et al. Early palliative care for patients with advanced cancer: a cluster-randomised controlled trial. *Lancet*. 2014;383(9930):1721-1730.

2.13-10.76; $P = .006$). Other measures of quality of life at the end of life ($P = .003$), symptoms ($P = .05$), and satisfaction with care ($P < .0001$) were superior in the early palliative care group at 4 months. Study caveats include a negative primary outcome with dual testing of multiple outcomes.

ASCO guidelines[10] recommend early palliative care involvement for patients with advanced cancer.

> You discharge the patient with close outpatient oncology and palliative care follow-up. A few months later, she presents with progressive malignant disease-causing worsening dyspnea. Working with the patient, her family, and her outpatient team, you enroll her in hospice, and she transitions her care mostly towards comfort. She finds great relief of her dyspnea from opioids you prescribe but is bothered by constipation despite low-dose senna. You wonder if docusate would be a good medication choice for her.

Is docusate effective for constipation in patients with advanced cancer?

No, docusate does not reduce constipation in this population.

This question was assessed in a 2008 nonrandomized, nonblinded, single-centered sequential cohort study among hospitalized cancer patients.[11] Patients were included if they were expected to require a bowel regimen and excluded if they had a previous bowel regimen they wished to continue, were unable to take oral medications, or had a colostomy or bowel obstruction. In the first cohort, 30 consecutive patients received an escalating docusate/senna protocol. The second cohort of 30 consecutive patients received an identical escalating regimen of senna but without any docusate (senna-only protocol). Patients in both cohorts were permitted to take other nonsenna/docusate bowel regimens as necessary. The primary outcomes were the proportion of days with ≥1 bowel movement and the proportion of patients with bowel

---

[10]Ferrell BR, et al. Integration of palliative care into standard oncology care: American Society of Clinical Oncology clinical practice guideline update. *J Clin Oncol*. 2016;35(1):96-112.
[11]Hawley PH, Byeon JJ. A comparison of sennosides-based bowel protocols with and without docusate in hospitalized patients with cancer. *J Palliat Med*. 2008;11(4):575-581.

movements on ≥40% and ≥50% of days. Secondary outcomes included the need for supplemental bowel regimens, cramping, and diarrhea. Patients were followed for up to 12 days, and most (80% in each group) were taking opiates.

There were no differences in any of the primary or secondary outcomes. In particular, the two cohorts had similar proportions of days with ≥1 bowel movement (49% under the docusate/senna protocol vs. 50% under the senna-only protocol; $P = .86$), proportion of patients with a bowel movement on ≥40% of days (60% vs. 80%; $P = .09$) and ≥50% of days (43.3% vs. 63.3%; $P = .12$), and use of additional bowel regimens (56.7% vs. 40%; $P = .19$). Study caveats include the nonrandomized, unblinded, and single-centered nature, small sample size, and selection bias from excluding patients who preferred their home bowel regimen.

In a 2013 double-blind, placebo-controlled trial, 74 patients at three Canadian inpatient hospice units were randomized to a regimen of senna plus docusate 200 mg po BID versus senna plus placebo.[12] Inclusion criteria included age ≥18 years of age and ability to take oral medications without swallowing problems. Patients were excluded if they had a gastrointestinal stoma or were already taking docusate as needed. Patients received sennoside 8.6 mg 1 to 3 tablets po QD to TID as well as either docusate 200 mg po BID or placebo. Additional open-label bowel regimens were permitted. The primary outcome was number of bowel movements per day. Other outcomes included "response" (defined as having a bowel movement on ≥50% of days), as well as patient report of strain with bowel movements and sensation of complete evacuation. Patients were followed for 10 days.

Most (>90%) patients in both groups used opiates daily and almost all (95%) had a primary malignant diagnosis. There was no difference between groups in the mean number of bowel movements per day (0.74 vs. 0.69/day; $P = .58$). There were no statistically significant differences in the rate of "response" (56% vs. 71%; P-value not reported), straining with bowel movements (32.5% vs. 25.0%; $P = .57$), or sense of complete evacuation (73.5% vs. 78.6%; $P = .77$). Study caveats include small sample size, questions about generalizability to a less terminally ill hospice population, and the possibility of selection bias due to the exclusion of patients already taking as needed docusate.

[12]Tarumi Y, et al. Randomized, double-blind, placebo-controlled trial of oral docusate in the management of constipation in hospice patients. *J Pain Symptom Manage.* 2013;45(1):2-13.

You increase the patient's dose of senna to 2 tablets tid, and she has resolution of her constipation and discomfort.

KEY LEARNING POINTS

1. PEG placement does not prolong life in patients with advanced dementia.
2. Family members who are invited to be present during a patient's CPR have lower subsequent rates of PTSD, depression, and complicated grief. Hospital family presence policies are not associated with harmful effects on CPR efforts or patient outcomes.
3. Early palliative care referral for advanced cancer can lead to improvements in quality of life for patients and short-term reductions in distress for their caregivers. In some cases, early palliative care is associated with longer survival.
4. Docusate is ineffective for constipation in patients with advanced cancer.

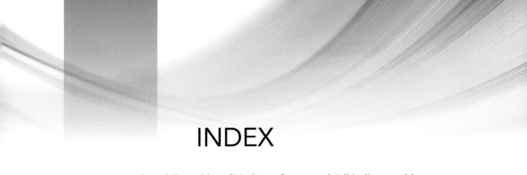

INDEX

Note: Page numbers followed by "f" indicate figures and "t" indicates tables.